7-MINUTE TOTAL-BODY WORKOUTS

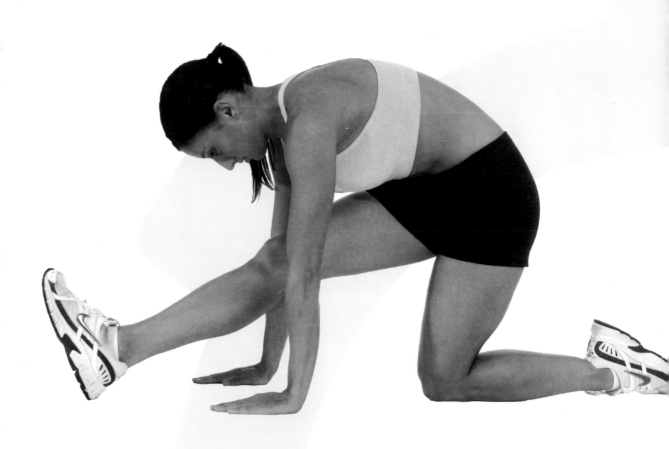

7-MINUTE
TOTAL-BODY
WORKOUTS

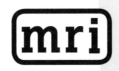

Michael Jerome

Published by Moseley Road Inc.

© Moseley Road Inc 2019

Created by Moseley Road Inc.
President: Sean Moore
Production Director: Adam Moore
Designer: Lisa Purcell
Layout Designer: Adam Moore
Editor: Finn Moore

ISBN: 9781626691599

Printed in China

Contents

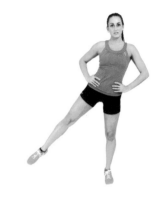
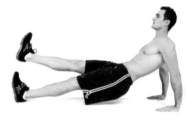
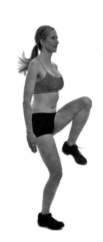

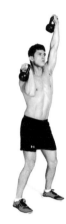

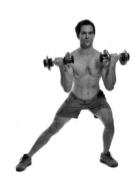

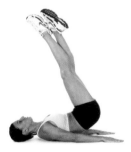

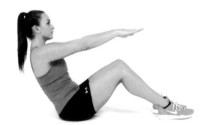

INTRODUCTION

TOTAL-BODY WORKOUTS: YOUR COMPLETE FITNESS REGIMEN

A Total-Body exercise is designed to incorporate several parts of the body, strengthening and toning your overall physique in a natural and consistent manner. Rather than targeting one part of your body at a time, Total-Body exercises allow your whole body to work as a single, efficient machine. Whether your goal is to lose weight, build muscle, or just improve your overall physical health, Total-Body exercises are the most efficient way to get started.

In this book, you'll find dozens of these Total-Body exercises, categorized into eight unique workout routines. Each routine has been carefully curated so that, when carried out to completion, you'll have put just about every muscle in your body through a vigorous workout. These routines can be as flexible as you need them to be; whether you're a beginner or whether you spend every day at the gym, you'll be able to use the workouts contained in this book to take your physical fitness to the next level.

7-MINUTE WORKOUTS: HOW TO USE THIS BOOK

This book is broken down into 8 workout routines, each featuring a different type of full body exercise. Within each routine, you'll find a selection of 12 unique exercises, complete with detailed step-by-step instructions, specific muscle groups that each exercise targets, and detailed tips to help you keep proper form and avoid injury.

By default, each workout is designed to take 7 minutes when performed as a single routine: this allows 30 seconds for each exercise, with a 5 second gap between each one. Moving steadily between each exercise without taking long breaks will help keep your heart rate up and keep your body active, and you should be able to fit one of these quick routines into even your busiest days.

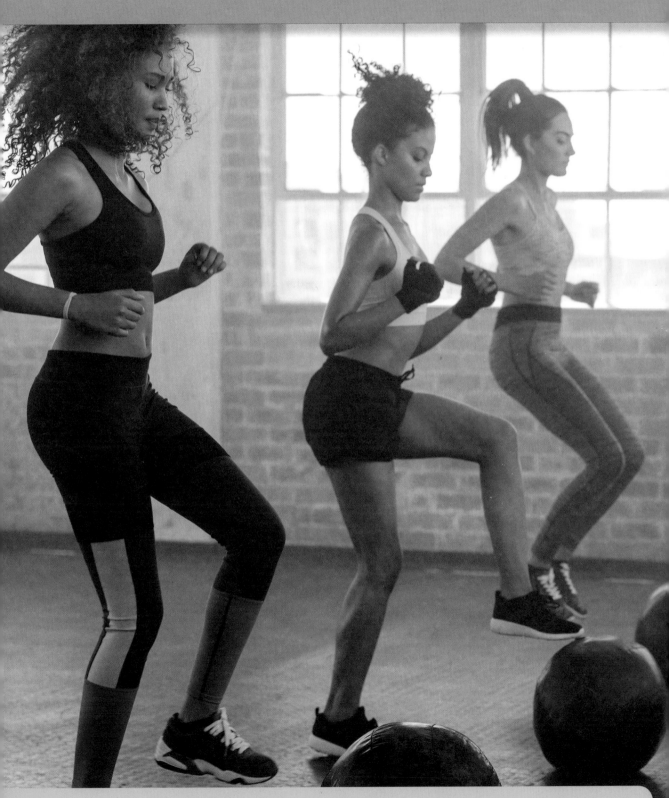

Of course, these workouts are only guidelines, and you should feel more than free to pick and choose, experiment, and figure out what kind of routine is best suited to your needs. Should you feel the need for a bit of a challenge, you might consider performing several sets of a routine, incorporating modifications to make the exercises more difficult, or even combining multiple workouts at once. If you're just getting started, or if you want to take things slowly, you may choose instead to take longer breaks between each exercise, or to simply focus on one exercise at a time. While the 7-minute method for each of these routines is designed to be both effective and accessible, you should always keep your own needs and goals in mind when designing your personal fitness routine.

WORKOUTS

This book is divided into 8 individual workout routines, each of which is modeled after a particular aspect of physical training. Although these routines can be performed in any order, either in tandem or independent of each other, you will also see great results by simply working through the book from start to finish. However, it's important to make sure that you perform these exercises properly—this will ensure that you benefit as much as possible from each exercise while reducing your risk of injuring yourself. With that said, here are some things to remember as you work through these exercises.

Workout 1: Stretching

Keep in mind: While stretching can be one of the least physically exerting types of exercise, it's important to remember proper form and technique. All of your movements should be smooth, gradual, and deliberate, and you should never force a stretch past your range of motion or to the point of pain or discomfort. Allowing yourself to complete a stretch to the best of your ability without pushing too hard is vital if you want to improve your overall flexibility and mobility.

Workout 2: Cardio

Keep in mind: You should always make sure to stay hydrated when you exercise, but that goes doubly for a cardio-heavy workout routine. Workouts that keep your heart rate up—running, swimming, and so on—burn up a lot of energy, and it's easy to get dehydrated if you're not careful.

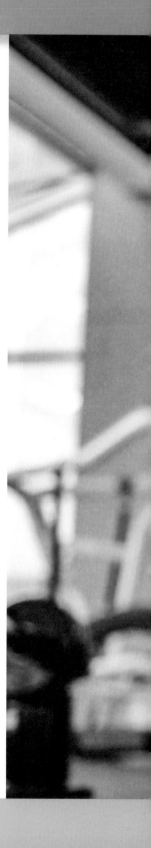

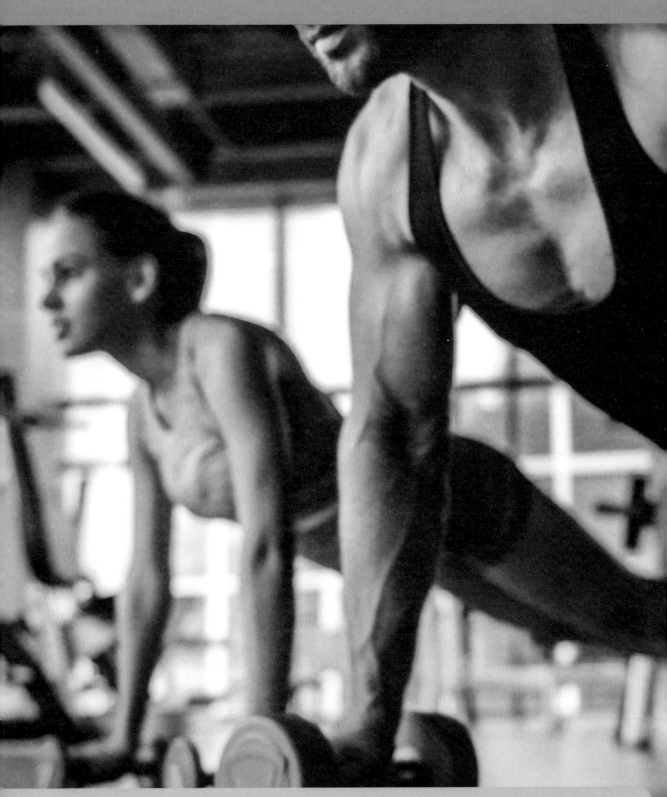

Workout 3: Weights

Keep in mind: It pays to understand the relationship between strength and endurance when it comes to lifting weights. Lifting an extremely heavy weight just a few times, for instance, is a good way to build muscle mass, allowing you to increase your maximum physical strength. Lifting a more manageable weight for several sets, on the other hand, helps build endurance and stamina, which allows you to work out for longer without getting tired. It's important to maintain a healthy balance between the two and to keep your goals in mind when picking out your weights.

Workout 4: Pilates-inspired

Keep in mind: Proper form is very important when performing these exercises. Because many of them are rather simple, small movements that require a great deal of muscle control to execute properly, it can be very tempting to "cheat" the exercise to make things a little easier. Avoid this whenever possible, as sloppy form both negates the value of the exercise and increase your risk of injury.

Workout 5: Yoga-inspired

Keep in mind: Yoga poses can be very difficult, and it's important to be aware of your body's limitations. Stretching requires you to put in some effort if you want to increase your flexibility, but forcing a stretch further than you're used to is a surefire way to injure yourself. If you can't quite complete a pose, do the best you can without causing pain, and try to get a little closer every day.

Workout 7: Upper Body Focus

Keep in mind: As always, proper form is vital whenever you're lifting heavy weights or performing a difficult stretch. Don't lock your joints or make any sudden, jerky movements when performing these exercises.

Workout 8: Lower Body

Keep in mind: Proper form is especially important for these exercises. You should take care to avoid overextending when performing exercises like squats, lunges, and heel-drops, and always keep your torso and hips correctly aligned when performing a squat or a lunge.

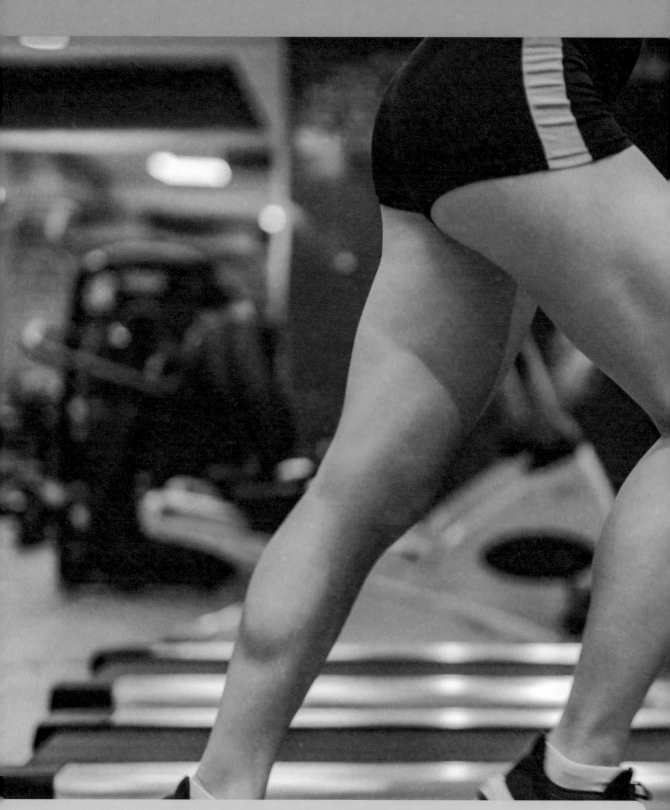

TOTAL-BODY ANATOMY

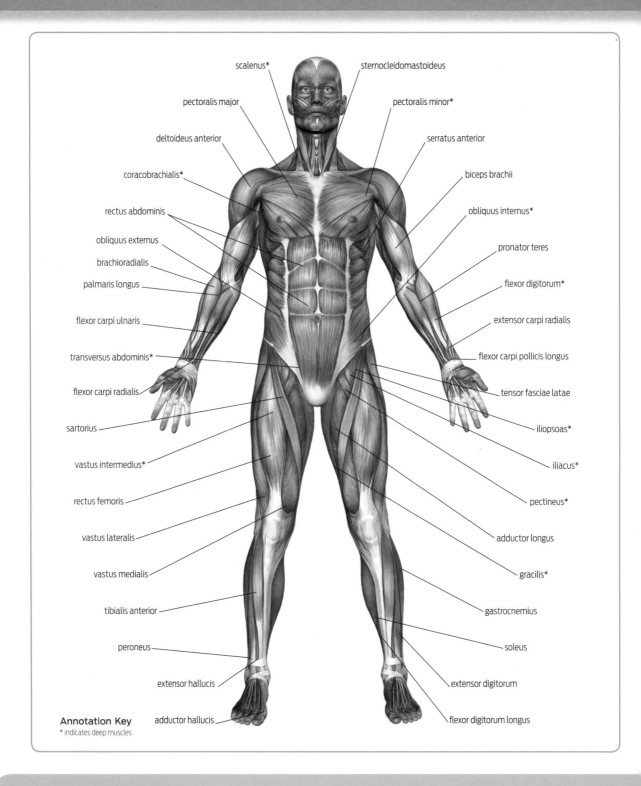

scalenus*

sternocleidomastoideus

pectoralis major

pectoralis minor*

deltoideus anterior

serratus anterior

coracobrachialis*

biceps brachii

rectus abdominis

obliquus internus*

obliquus externus

pronator teres

brachioradialis

palmaris longus

flexor digitorum*

flexor carpi ulnaris

extensor carpi radialis

transversus abdominis*

flexor carpi pollicis longus

flexor carpi radialis

tensor fasciae latae

sartorius

iliopsoas*

vastus intermedius*

iliacus*

rectus femoris

pectineus*

vastus lateralis

adductor longus

vastus medialis

gracilis*

tibialis anterior

gastrocnemius

peroneus

soleus

extensor hallucis

extensor digitorum

Annotation Key
* indicates deep muscles

adductor hallucis

flexor digitorum longus

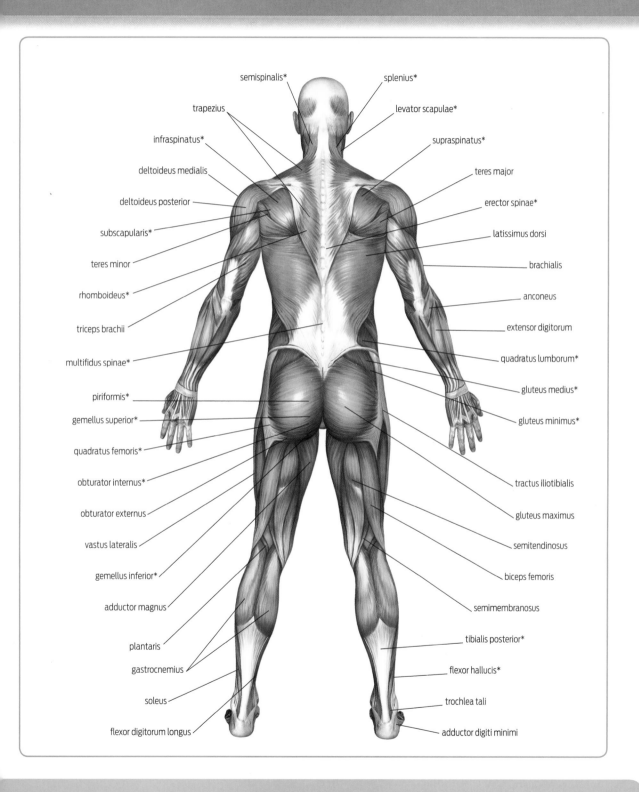

semispinalis*

splenius*

trapezius

levator scapulae*

infraspinatus*

supraspinatus*

deltoideus medialis

teres major

deltoideus posterior

erector spinae*

subscapularis*

latissimus dorsi

teres minor

brachialis

rhomboideus*

anconeus

triceps brachii

extensor digitorum

multifidus spinae*

quadratus lumborum*

piriformis*

gluteus medius*

gemellus superior*

gluteus minimus*

quadratus femoris*

obturator internus*

tractus iliotibialis

obturator externus

gluteus maximus

vastus lateralis

semitendinosus

gemellus inferior*

biceps femoris

adductor magnus

semimembranosus

plantaris

tibialis posterior*

gastrocnemius

flexor hallucis*

soleus

trochlea tali

flexor digitorum longus

adductor digiti minimi

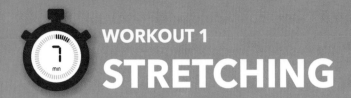
1 Upper-Back / Shoulder Stretch

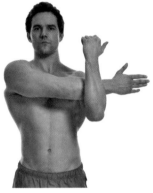

2 Biceps-Pecs Stretch

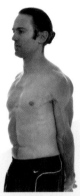

3 Triceps Stretch

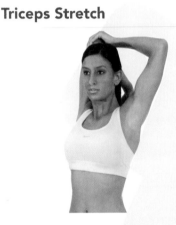

4 Straddle Abductor Stretch

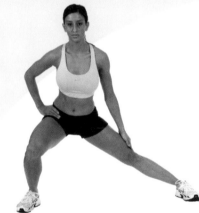

5 Hip Flexor and Hamstrings Stretch

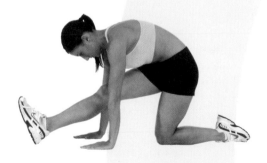

6 Wall-Assisted Chest Stretch

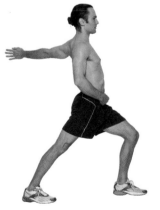

This workout is your best bet in terms of warming up, cooling down, and keeping yourself flexible and limber. You can perform these stretches just about anywhere, as long as you have some free floor space and comfortable clothes that won't restrict your movement. Hold each stretch for up to 30 seconds.

7 Couch Stretch

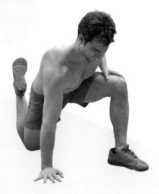

8 Lower-Back and Hip Stretch

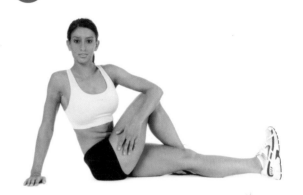

9 Seated Leg Cradle

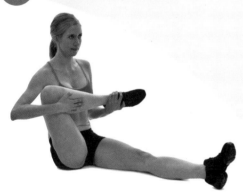

10 Spine Stretch

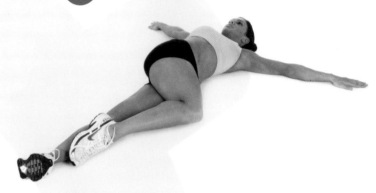

11 Piriformis Stretch

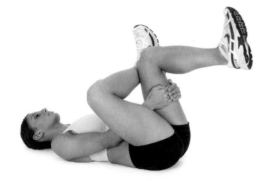

12 Kneeling Lat Stretch

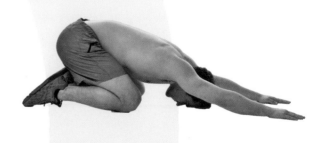

1

TIME ELAPSED

• 30 sec

BEST FOR

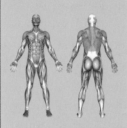

FRONT BACK

• Upper back
• Shoulders

UPPER-BACK / SHOULDER STRETCH

1 Stand up straight with one arm drawn across your chest.

2 Keep your other arm bent and pointed upward while linking with the extended arm.

3 Gently pull your extended arm further across your chest.

4 Hold for several seconds, then switch sides.

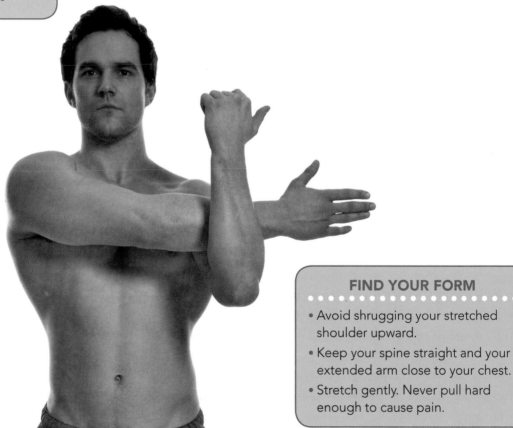

FIND YOUR FORM

• Avoid shrugging your stretched shoulder upward.
• Keep your spine straight and your extended arm close to your chest.
• Stretch gently. Never pull hard enough to cause pain.

BEST FOR

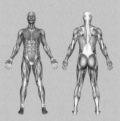

FRONT   BACK

• Biceps
• Chest

BICEPS-PECS STRETCH

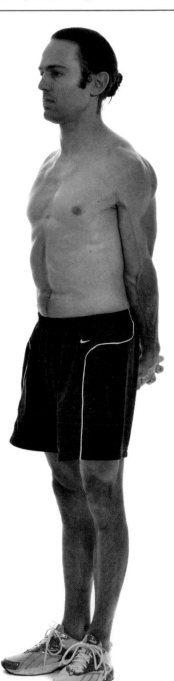

❶ Stand with your feet shoulder-width apart and your knees relaxed.

❷ Link your hands together behind your back.

❸ Extend your arms downward, simultaneously twisting your palms inward.

FIND YOUR FORM

• •

• Avoid allowing your chest to dip forward.
• Keep your shoulders pressed downward and back.

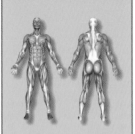

FRONT   BACK

• Shoulders
• Triceps

TRICEPS STRETCH

① Stand in a neutral position, keeping your neck, torso, and shoulders straight. Raise your right arm and bend it behind your head. Keeping your shoulders relaxed, grasp your raised elbow with your left hand and gently pull back.

② Continue to pull your elbow back until you feel the stretch on the underside of your arm.

③ Repeat with the opposite arm.

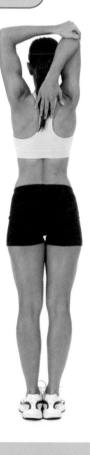

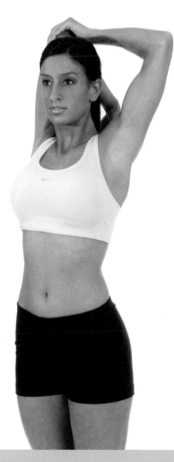

FIND YOUR FORM

• Avoid leaning backward.
• Keep your dropped elbow close to the side of your head.

4

• 2 min

BEST FOR

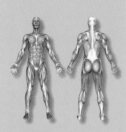

FRONT   BACK

• Inner thighs
• Hamstrings

STRADDLE ABDUCTOR STRETCH

① Stand with your feet wider than shoulder width apart and bend your knees.

② Place your hands on your knees and bend at your hips, keeping your back straight and your shoulders slightly forward.

③ Keeping your torso in the same position and your hips behind your heels, shift your weight to the right, bending your right knee while extending your left leg.

④ Hold, release, and repeat on other side.

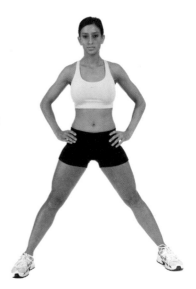

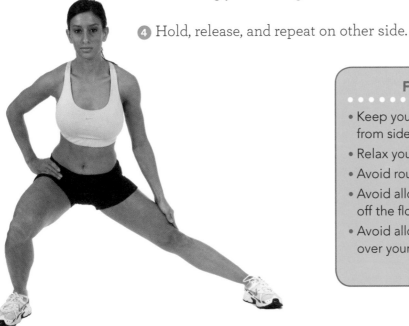

FIND YOUR FORM

• Keep your torso aligned as you move from side to side.
• Relax your neck and shoulders.
• Avoid rounding your spine.
• Avoid allowing your feet to shift or lift off the floor.
• Avoid allowing your knees to extend over your toes while bending.

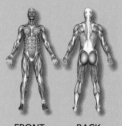

FRONT   BACK

• Hip flexors
• Hamstrings

HIP FLEXOR AND HAMSTRINGS STRETCH

① Kneel on the ground with your right foot flat on the floor in front of you. Extend your back foot so that the top of your foot rests on the floor.

② Bring your torso forward, extending your back leg and bending your right knee so that your knee shifts toward your toes. Keeping your torso upright, press your right hip forward and downward to create a stretch over the front of your thigh. Extend your arms above your head, keeping your shoulders relaxed.

③ Bring your arms down and move your hips backward. Extend your right leg until only your heel rest son the floor and lean your upper body forward. Place your hands on either side of your straight leg for support.

④ Hold, then repeat with the other leg.

FIND YOUR FORM

- Avoid extending your front knee too far over your foot.
- Keep your shoulders, hips, and knees aligned.
- Keep your shoulders and neck relaxed.
- Move slowly and smoothly, avoiding sudden motions.

CHALLENGE YOURSELF

During the backward movement, raise your back knee off the floor and straighten your back leg. Keep your hands on the floor.

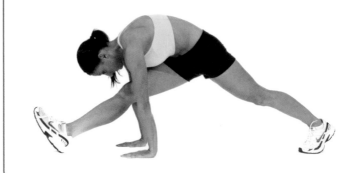

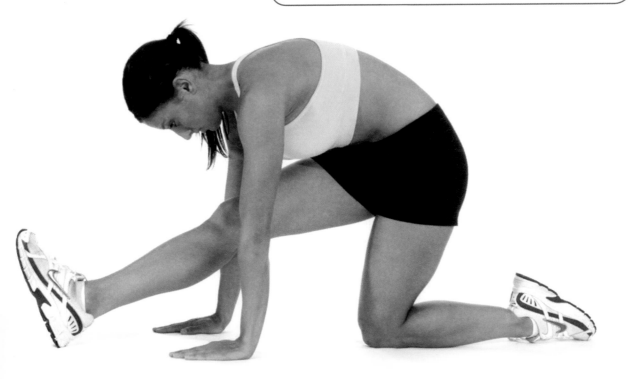

TIME ELAPSED

• 3 min

BEST FOR

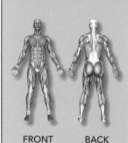

FRONT   BACK

• Chest
• Biceps

WALL-ASSISTED CHEST STRETCH

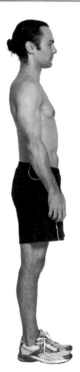

① Stand next to a wall with the wall on the left side of your body.

② Extend your left arm behind yourself and press your palm flat against the wall.

③ Lunge slowly forward with your left foot, keeping your palm on the wall for support.

④ Remain facing forward as you stretch, keeping your head, shoulders, and hips aligned.

⑤ Hold, and then return to the starting position, turn so that the wall is on your right, and repeat.

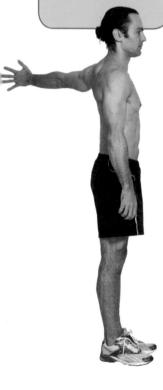

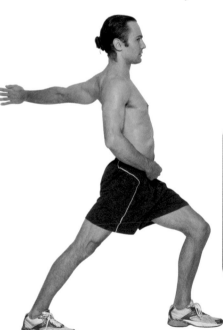

FIND YOUR FORM

• Avoid rotating your torso and chest inward toward the wall.
• Keep your shoulders pressed downward and back.
• Keep your upper arm shoulder level and parallel to the floor.

BEST FOR

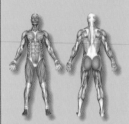

FRONT   BACK

• Gluteal muscles
• Thighs
• Hip flexors

COUCH STRETCH

1 Kneel on the floor. Bend the knee of your back leg and rest your shin against the wall behind you so that only your knee touches the floor.

2 Arch and relax your back, holding the position. Keep your other foot flat on the floor, supporting yourself with one hand on the ground and one on your front thigh.

3 Switch sides, and then repeat on the other leg.

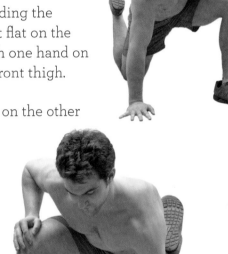

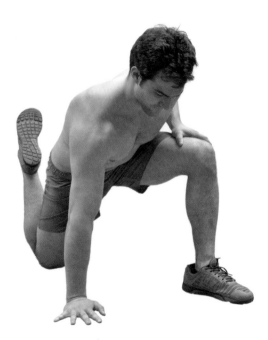

FIND YOUR FORM

• Avoid overextending your back leg.
• Keep your front foot and knee in line.
• Arch and relax your back to engage your muscles.

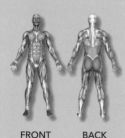
LOWER-BACK AND HIP STRETCH

① Sit with your left leg extended straight in front of you and bend your right knee. Cross your bent knee over the straight leg and keep your right foot flat on the floor.

② Wrap your left arm around the bent knee. Pull gently and rotate your torso toward your bent knee, placing your right hand on the floor for stability.

③ Keeping your hips steady, rotate your upper body as you pull your knee slightly in the other direction.

④ Hold. Slowly release and repeat on the other side.

FIND YOUR FORM

• Avoid rounding your torso.
• Avoid lifting the foot of your bent leg off the floor.
• Avoid straining your neck as you rotate.
• Keep your neck and shoulders relaxed.
• Apply even pressure to your leg with your active hand.

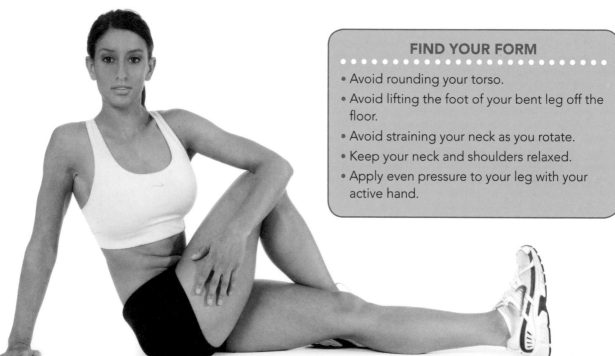

BEST FOR

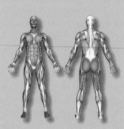

FRONT   BACK

• Gluteal muscles
• Hamstrings

SEATED LEG CRADLE

① Sit on the floor with your legs extended in front of you.

② Lift one knee toward your torso, supporting your calf and ankle with both hands, and gently bring your calf and ankle towards your chest.

③ Gently pull your leg into your torso until your heel is about a foot from your chest. Hold.

④ Switch sides, and then repeat with the other leg.

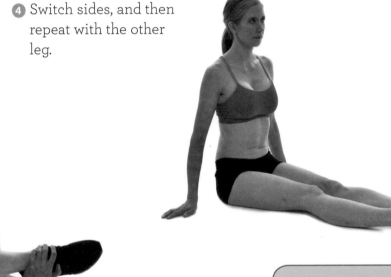

FIND YOUR FORM

• Avoid aggressively pulling on your leg.
• Breathe evenly.
• Use your hands to assist the stretch, but let most of the work come from your glutes and thighs.

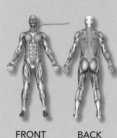
SPINE STRETCH

1 Lie on your back. Extend your left leg and bend your right leg, resting your right foot flat on top of your left shin. Extend your arms in line with your shoulders and keep your palms pressed to the floor.

2 Keeping both shoulders on the floor, slowly bring your right leg across your body. Stretch only as far as your shoulders will allow without one of them rising from the floor.

3 Hold, slowly return to the starting position, and repeat on the other side.

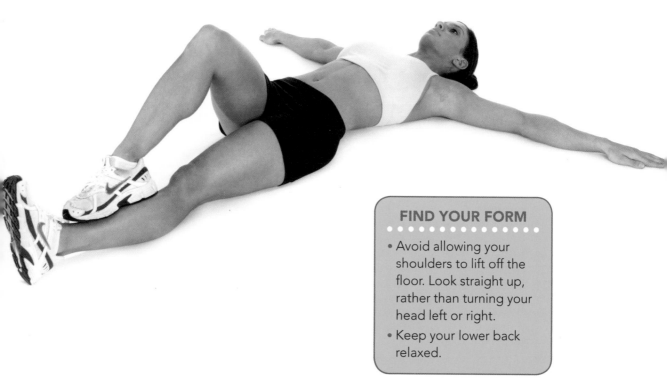

FIND YOUR FORM

• Avoid allowing your shoulders to lift off the floor. Look straight up, rather than turning your head left or right.

• Keep your lower back relaxed.

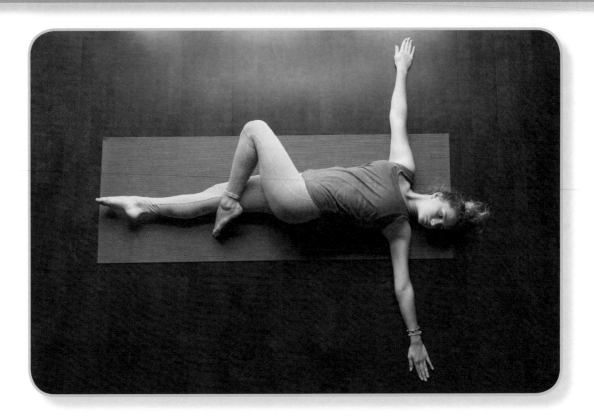

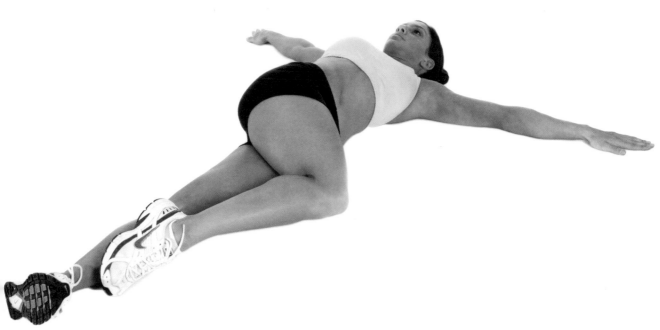

TIME ELAPSED

• 5 min, 30 sec

BEST FOR

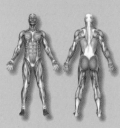

FRONT   BACK

• Gluteal muscles
• Lower Back
• Hips

PIRIFORMIS STRETCH

❶ Lie on your back with your knees bent and your feet flat on the floor.

❷ Lift your left leg and place your left ankle over your right knee. Wrap both hands around your right thigh.

❸ Gently pull your right thigh toward your chest and hold for a few seconds. Slowly return to the starting position.

❹ Repeat on the other side.

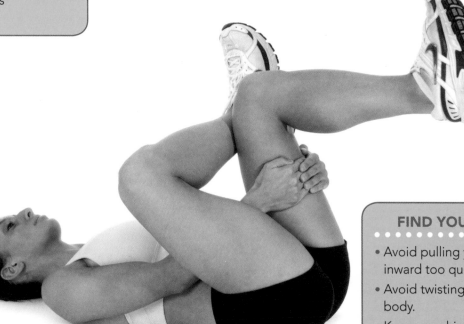

FIND YOUR FORM

• Avoid pulling your leg inward too quickly.
• Avoid twisting your lower body.
• Keep your hips relaxed and in line with your shoulders.
• Keep your head and shoulders on the floor.

BEST FOR

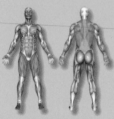

FRONT   BACK

• Back
• Thighs

KNEELING LAT STRETCH

1. Kneel in front of a couch or other solid surface with your back leg bent and your shin and foot placed against the couch and the other leg forward with your foot flat.

2. Arch your back, and hold for 10 seconds.

3. Relax your back, switch sides, and repeat on the other side.

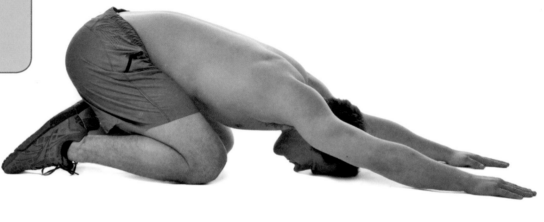

FIND YOUR FORM

• Extend your back to the limit of your range of motion, but no further.

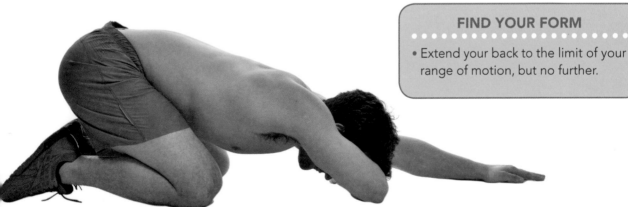

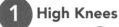
1 High Knees

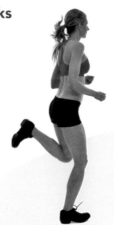

2 Butt Kicks

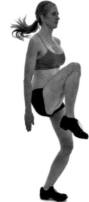

3 Bench Dip

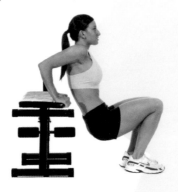

4 Skater's Lunge

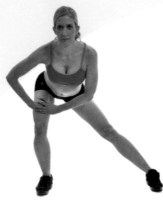

5 Power Punch

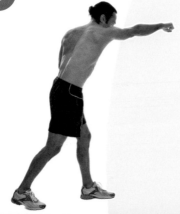

6 Uppercut

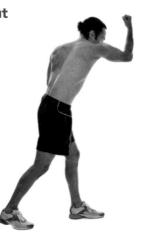

Cardio is the ideal type of exercise for anyone looking to lose weight, maintain your metabolism, and improve your overall heart health. These exercises are designed to keep your heart rate up and your blood pumping, and the more consistently you can perform them, the better results you'll start to see. Perform each exercise for 30 seconds with only a 5-second rest for an intensive HIIT workout.

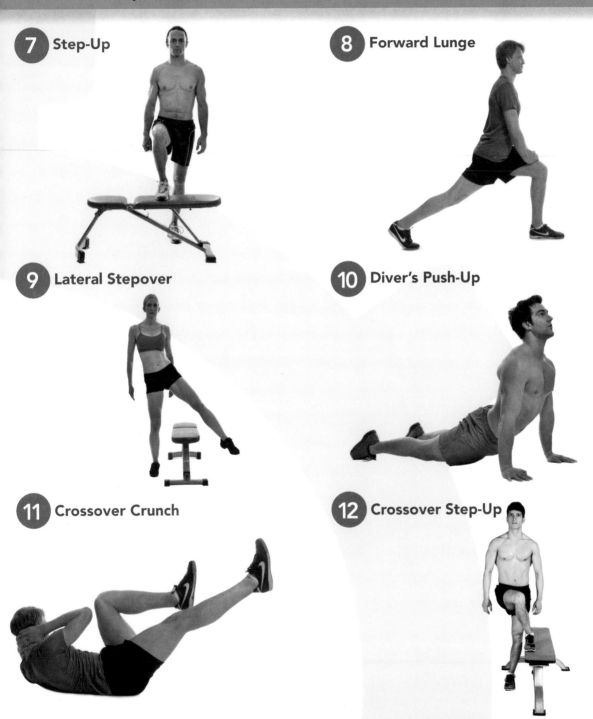

7 Step-Up

8 Forward Lunge

9 Lateral Stepover

10 Diver's Push-Up

11 Crossover Crunch

12 Crossover Step-Up

TIME ELAPSED

- 30 sec

BEST FOR

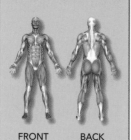

FRONT   BACK

- Calves
- Glutes
- Thighs

HIGH KNEES

1. Stand tall with your hands either on your hips or down by your sides.

2. Raise up one knee as high as you are able, and then return to the starting position.

3. Alternate legs while increasing your speed as you jog in place.

FIND YOUR FORM

- Build up in speed as you go.
- Push off from your entire foot.
- Avoid pushing solely off your toes.

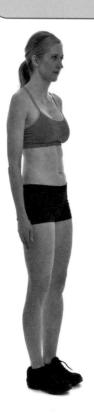

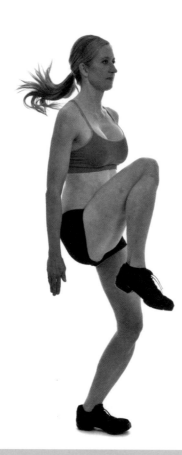

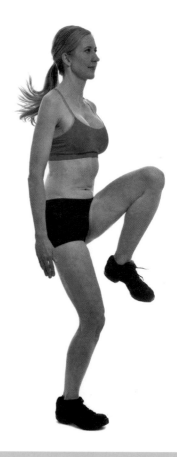

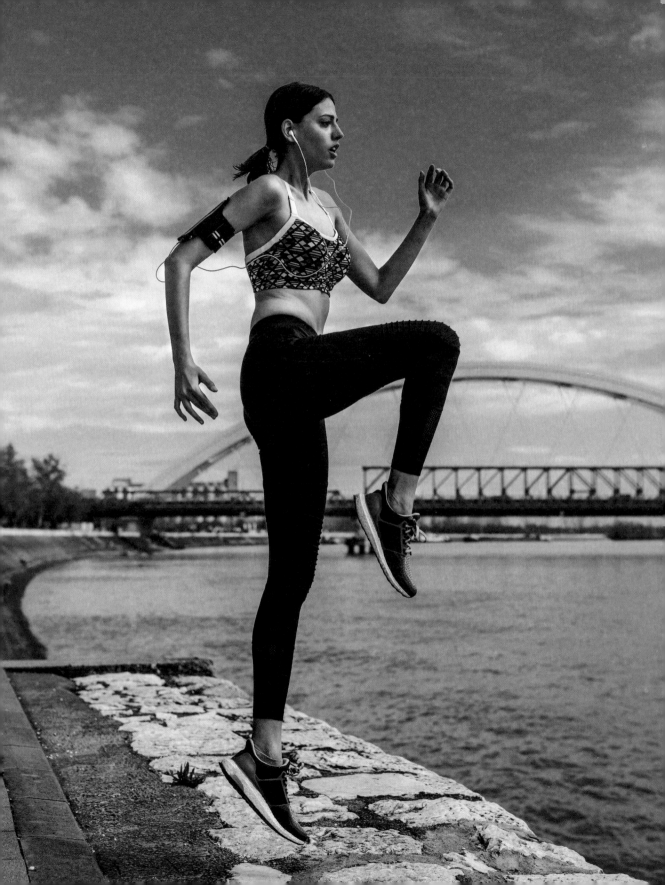

2

TIME ELAPSED

• 1 min

BEST FOR

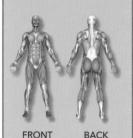

FRONT   BACK

• Calves
• Glutes
• Thighs

BUTT KICKS

① Begin in a standing position, and then jog in place.

② Kick your heels up high toward your glutes.

③ Continue jogging in place, lifting your heels high and increasing your speed as you go.

CHALLENGE YOURSELF

Weighted ankle straps will add a degree of difficulty to this exercise. As you become more adept at performing this, try to increase the speed of your kicks.

FIND YOUR FORM

• Build up speed as you jog in place.
• Bend your knees when placing your feet back on the floor to reduce impact.

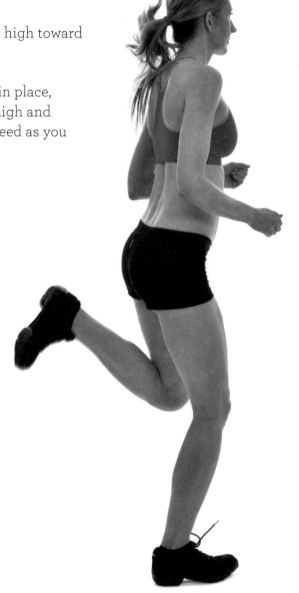

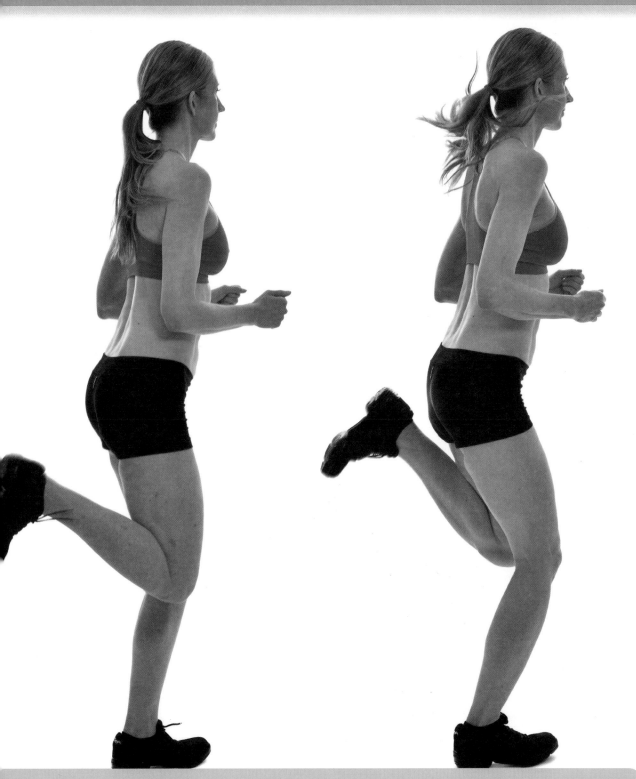

TIME ELAPSED

- 1 min, 30 sec

BEST FOR

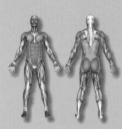

FRONT   BACK

- Triceps
- Shoulder
- Core

BENCH DIP

① Sit up tall near the front of a flat bench. Place your hands beside your hips, wrapping your fingers over the front edge of the bench.

② Extend your legs in front of you slightly and place your feet flat on the floor.

③ Scoot off the edge of the bench until your knees align directly above your feet and your torso will be able to clear the bench as you dip down.

④ Bending your elbows directly behind you, without splaying them out to the sides, lower your torso until your elbows make a 90-degree angle.

⑤ Press into the bench, raising your body back to the starting position.

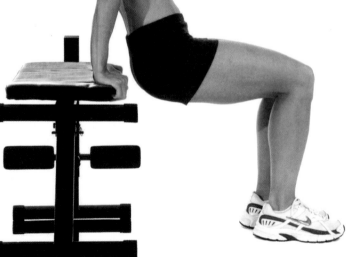

FIND YOUR FORM

- Keep your body close to the bench.
- Keep your back relaxed.
- Avoid allowing your shoulders to lift toward your ears.
- Avoid moving your feet.
- Avoid rounding your back at your hips.

CHALLENGE YOURSELF

Keeping your knees squeezed together, perform the dips with one leg lifted straight out, parallel to the floor.

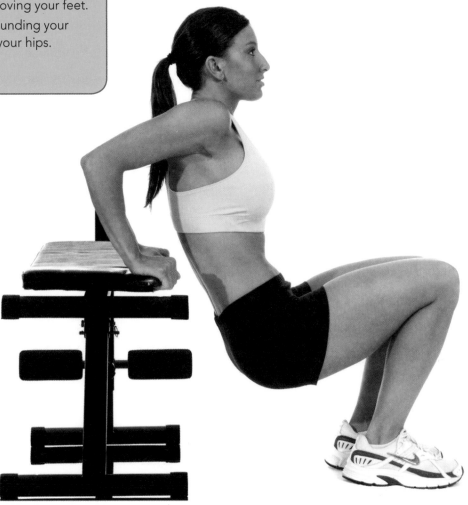

4

TIME ELAPSED

• 2 min

BEST FOR

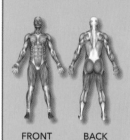

FRONT   BACK

• Glutes
• Hamstrings
• Thighs

SKATER'S LUNGE

1 Stand with your legs spaced wider than shoulder-width apart and your toes pointing forward.

2 Slide to your side into a side lunge as you bend forward slightly, with your hands placed on your thigh, and then move in the opposite direction.

3 Slide back and forth, alternating sides.

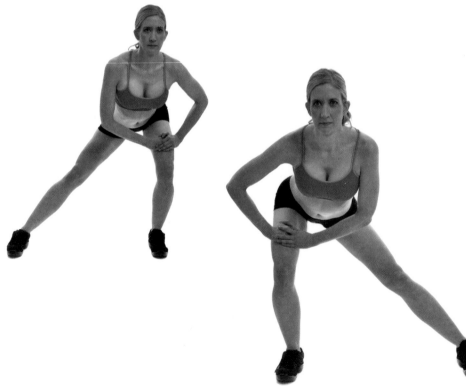

FIND YOUR FORM

- Push through the heel to drive the exercise.
- Move with control, keeping a steady, quick pace.
- Avoid hyperextending your knee past your toes.

CHALLENGE YOURSELF

Try using dumbbells as you lean from side to side.

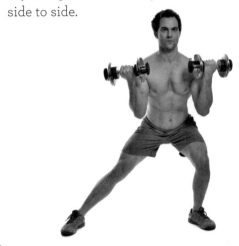

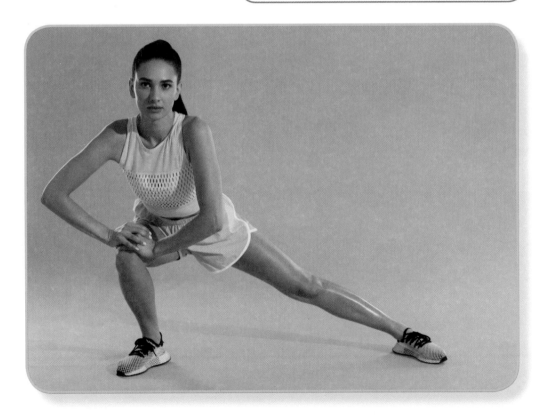

5

TIME ELAPSED

• 2 min, 30 sec

BEST FOR

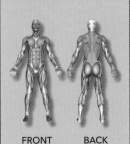

FRONT　　BACK

• Back
• Shoulders

POWER PUNCH

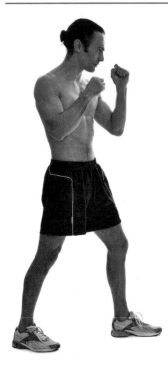

1 Stand with your feet shoulder width apart and one leg placed slightly in front of the other, placing most of your weight on your back leg. Keep your elbows in and raise your fists up.

2 Transferring your weight to your front leg, punch straight in front of you with the fist closest to your body as you turn your torso in to lend power to the punch.

3 Punch 10 times, and then reverse sides, switching both arms and legs.

FIND YOUR FORM

• Maintain a steady pace.
• Rotate your torso to drive the movement.
• Keep your fists up.

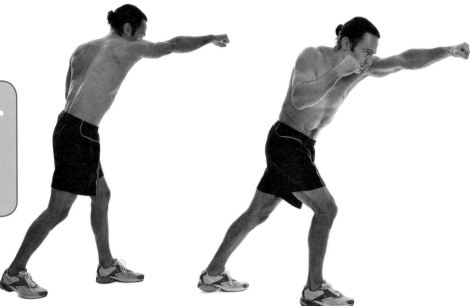

TIME ELAPSED

• 3 min

BEST FOR

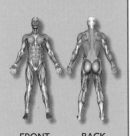

FRONT   BACK

• Back
• Shoulders

UPPERCUT

1 Stand with your feet shoulder width apart and one leg placed slightly in front of the other, placing most of your weight on your back leg. Keep your elbows in and raise your fists up.

2 Keeping your elbows in, raise your fists up and punch upward toward the sky as you rotate your torso and transfer most of your weight to your front foot.

3 Alternate sides every few punches, switching both arms and legs.

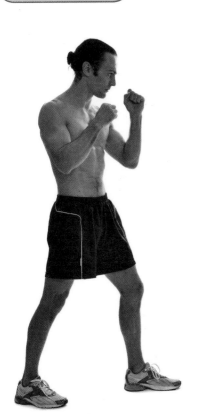

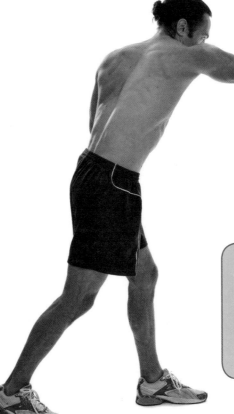

FIND YOUR FORM

• Rotate your torso to drive the movement.
• Avoid overextending your active arm.

BEST FOR

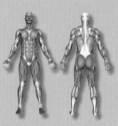

FRONT   BACK

• Glutes
• Hamstrings
• Thighs

STEP-UP

1 Begin in a standing position behind a flat bench or elevated platform and place your right foot on it.

2 Step up onto the bench until your left leg is straight, using your right hamstring and glute to complete the movement. Lower your left leg and repeat.

3 Switch starting position with your left leg on the bench and repeat on the other side.

CHALLENGE YOURSELF

Try doing the exercise while holding dumbbells, kettlebells, or a heavy plate held at chest height. Adding weight to any exercise will automatically increase its effectiveness..

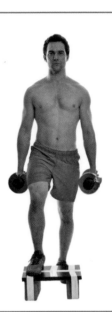

FIND YOUR FORM

• Push through the working heel, keep that foot planted.

• Avoid hyperextending your knee past your toes.

• Move slowly and deliberately.

TIME ELAPSED

• 4 min

BEST FOR

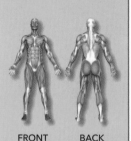

FRONT   BACK

• Thighs
• Glutes
• Calves
• Hips

FORWARD LUNGE

1 Stand with your legs and feet parallel and shoulder width apart, and your knees bent very slightly. Tuck your pelvis slightly forwards, lift your chest and press your shoulders down and back.

2 Bend your left knee, and step your right leg back behind your body, extending it straight.

3 Place your palms on your knee and hold.

4 Release the stretch, switch legs and repeat.

FIND YOUR FORM

• Keep your back leg extended in line with your hips to form one long straight line.
• Keep your knee directly above your ankle.
• Breathe evenly as you stretch.
• Avoid dropping the elevated arm behind you - look for both arms to remain on the same plane.

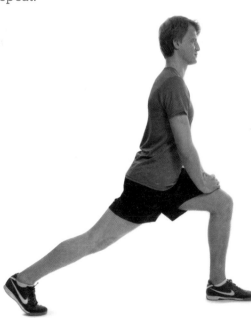

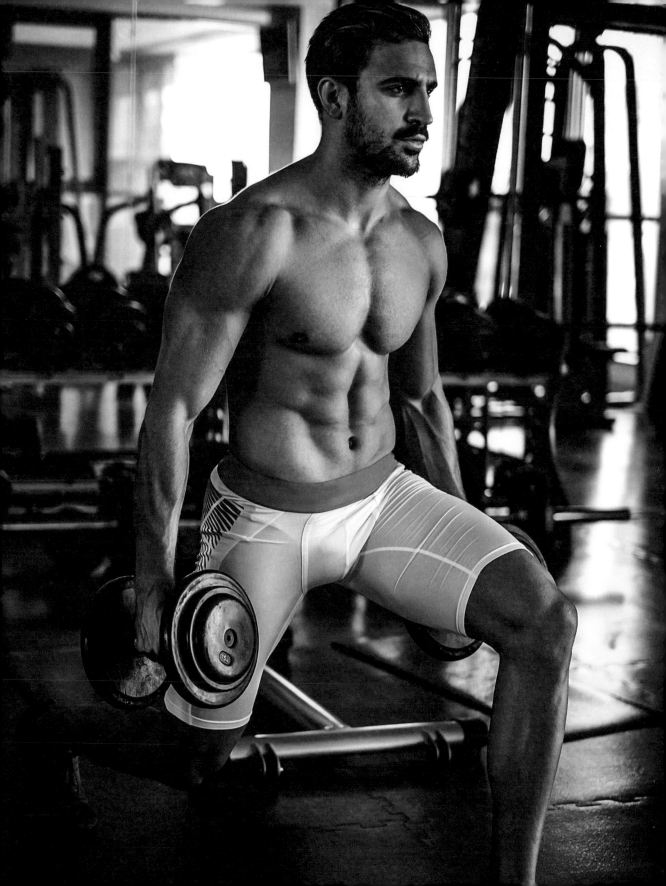

BEST FOR

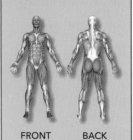

FRONT   BACK

• Glutes
• Hamstrings
• Thighs

LATERAL STEPOVER

1 Stand next to a flat bench.

2 Raise the knee of the leg closest to the bench, and then lower it down on the opposite side of the bench.

3 Lift the opposite leg to meet the other, bringing your feet together.

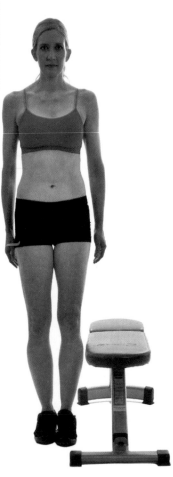

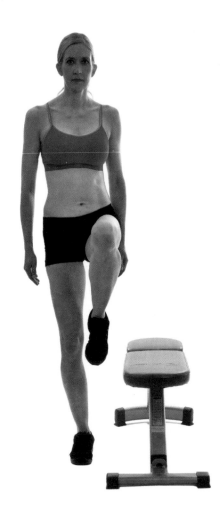

FIND YOUR FORM

• • • • • • • • • • • • • • • • • • •

- Move slowly and evenly.
- Push through your heel to drive the movement.
- Avoid allowing your knees to hyperextend past your feet.

CHALLENGE YOURSELF

Depending on your level of fitness, you may want to start out with a lower obstacle to step over, and gradually build up to a bench, and maybe even an inclined bench eventually.

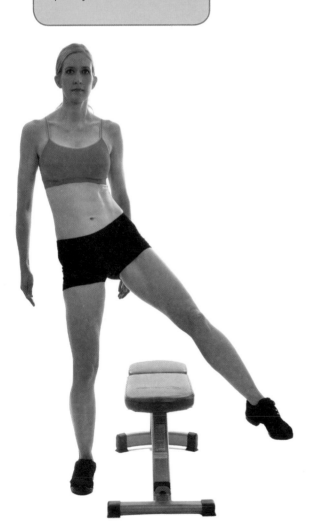

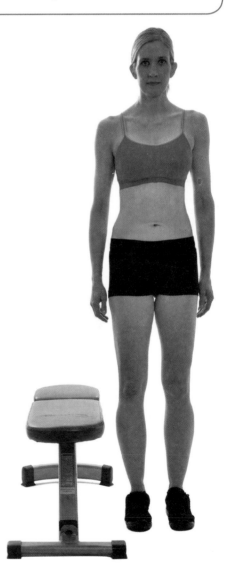

BEST FOR

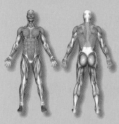

FRONT   BACK

• Shoulders
• Chest
• Back
• Abdominals

DIVER'S PUSH-UP

❶ Begin in the Downward-Facing Dog position.

❷ With a controlled movement, swoop your hips toward the floor while simultaneously raising your chest.

❸ Continue rising upward until you're looking toward the ceiling and your back is arched.

❹ Lower your torso back down and the repeat the entire sequence.

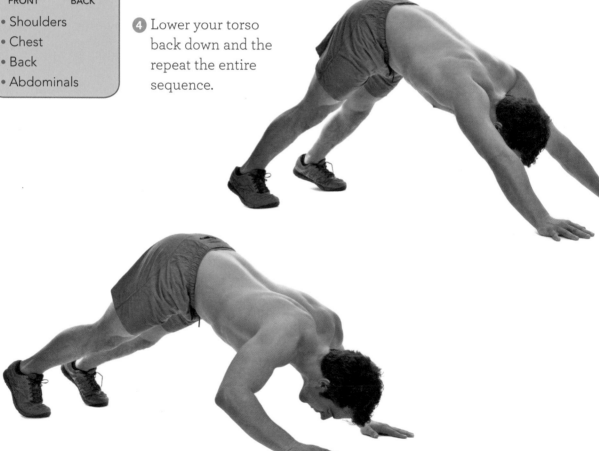

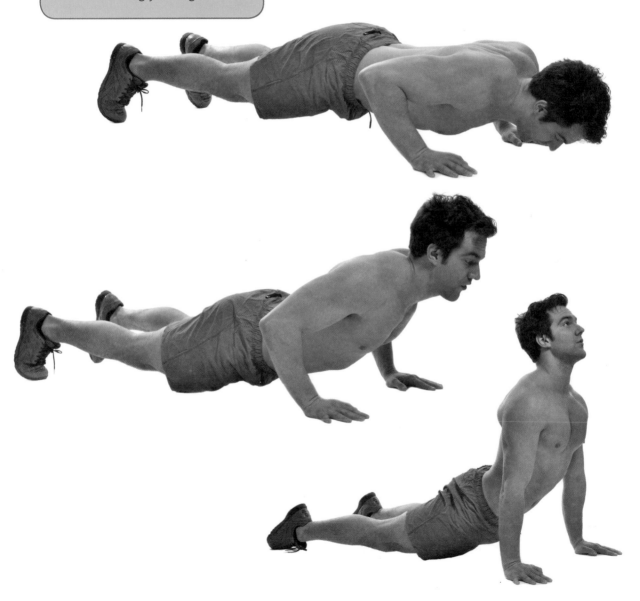

FIND YOUR FORM

- Press your forearms and palms firmly to the floor.
- Move slowly and deliberately.
- Avoid bending your legs.

TIME ELAPSED

• 5 min, 30 sec

BEST FOR

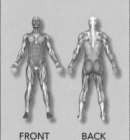

FRONT   BACK

• Core
• Abs

CROSSOVER CRUNCH

1 Bring your hands behind your head and lift your legs off the floor into a tabletop position, so that your thighs and calves form a 90-degree angle.

2 Roll up with your torso, reaching your right elbow to your left knee and extending the right leg in front of you. Imagine pulling your shoulder blades off the floor and twisting from your ribs and oblique muscles.

3 Alternate sides. Repeat sequence six times.

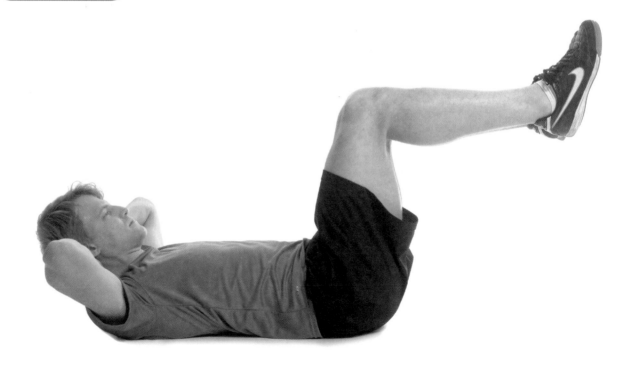

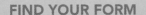

FIND YOUR FORM

- Elongate your neck.
- Lift your chin away from your chest.
- Keep both hips stable on the floor.
- Avoid pulling with your hands.
- Avoid arching your back.

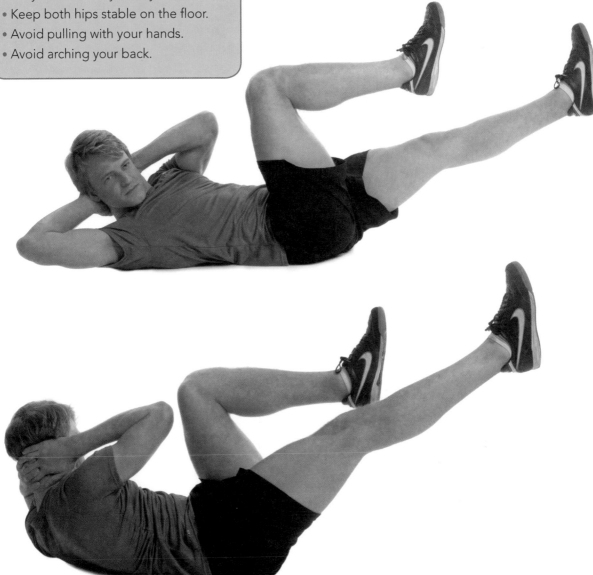

CROSSOVER STEP-UP

BEST FOR

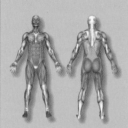

FRONT   BACK

• Thighs
• Hamstrings
• Glutes
• Core

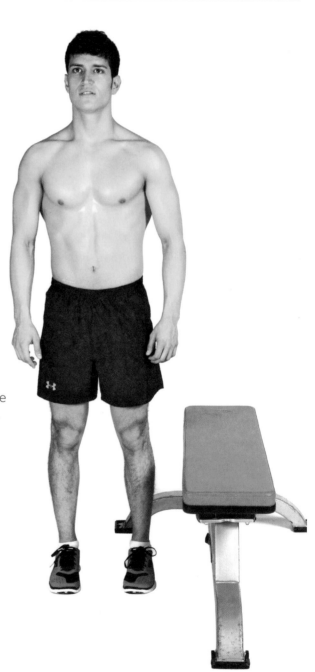

1 Stand to the right of a bench.

2 Cross your right leg in front of your left and step onto the bench. Push through the stabilized right heel on the bench to raise yourself up.

3 Bring the left leg up on to the bench, perform the motion in reverse to step down. Repeat, alternating legs every few steps.

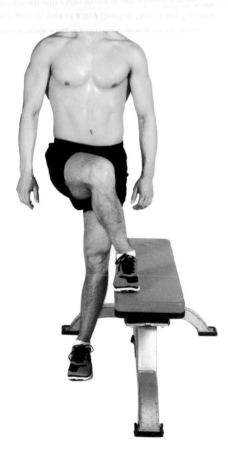

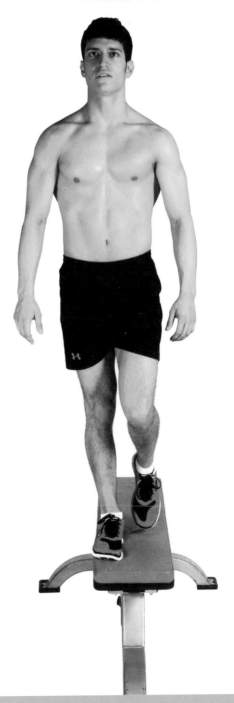

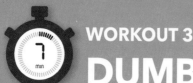
1 **Dumbbell Deadlift**

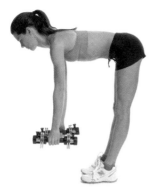

2 **Triceps Extension**

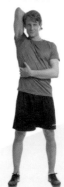

3 **Alternating Dumbbell Curl**

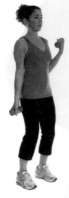

4 **Single-Leg Deadlift**

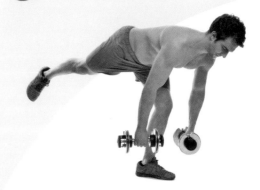

5 **Dumbbell Lunge**

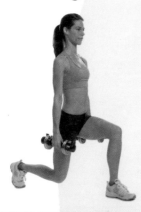

6 **Lateral Shoulder Raise**

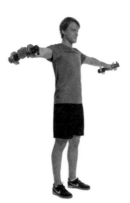

This workout routine is intended to build strength and muscle mass. While many workouts are geared towards strength training, many also tend to focus too much on the upper body. These exercises will help you strengthen your arms, legs, back, and chest in tandem, which should allow you to maintain a more even and powerful physique.

7 Shoulder Raise and Pull

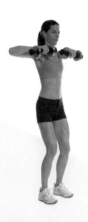

8 Dumbbell Upright Row

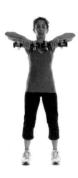

9 Sumo Squat

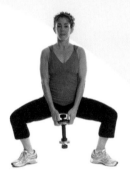

10 Dumbbell Calf Raise

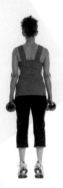

11 Lunge with Dumbbell Upright Row

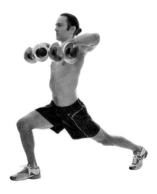

12 Seated Alternating Dumbbell Press

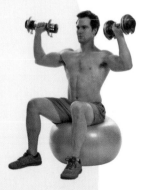

TIME ELAPSED

• 30 sec

BEST FOR

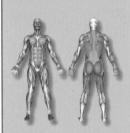

FRONT   BACK

• Glutes
• Hamstrings
• Back

DUMBBELL DEADLIFT

1 Stand upright, feet planted about shoulder-width apart.

2 Hold your arms slightly out in front of your thighs with a hand weight or dumbbell in each hand. Your knees should be relaxed and your rear pushed slightly outwards.

3 Keeping your back flat, hinge at the hips and bend forwards as you lower the dumbbells towards the floor. You should feel a stretch in the backs of your legs.

4 With control, raise your upper body back to starting position and repeat.

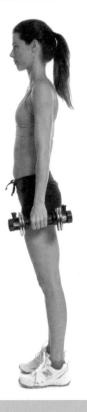

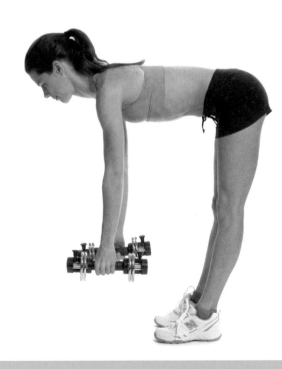

FIND YOUR FORM

• Maintain the straight line of your back.
• Keep your neck straight.
• Avoid allowing your lower back to sag or arch.

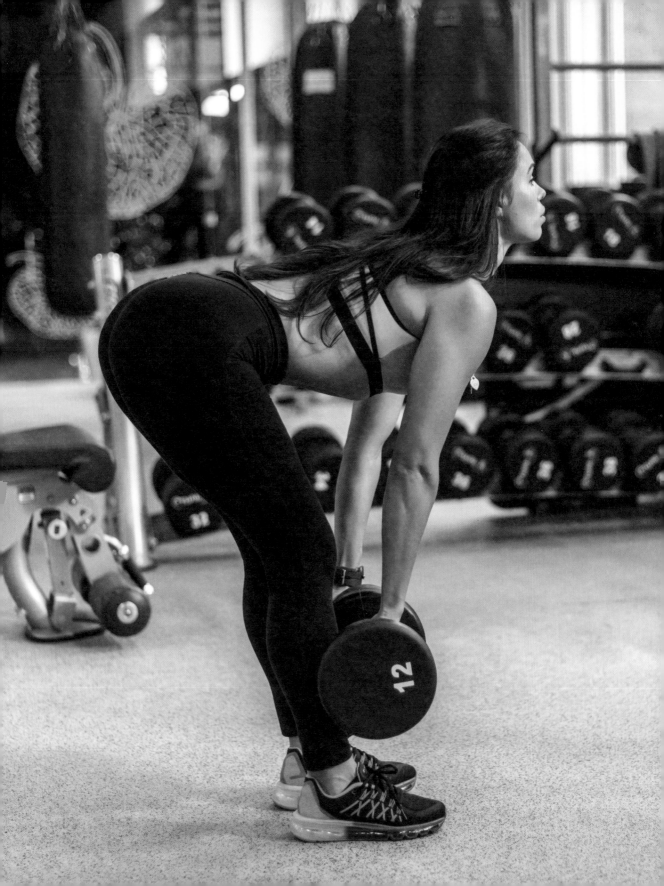

2

TIME ELAPSED

• 1 min

BEST FOR

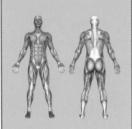

FRONT   BACK

• Upper Arms
• Triceps

TRICEPS EXTENSION

1 Stand with your legs and feet parallel and shoulder width apart, grasping a dumbbell or hand weight in your right hand. Position the dumbbell over your head with your arm extended and angled slightly backward.

2 Lower the dumbbell behind your neck or shoulder while maintaining your upper arm's vertical position.

3 Extend your arm until straight.

4 Return to starting position and repeat on the opposite side.

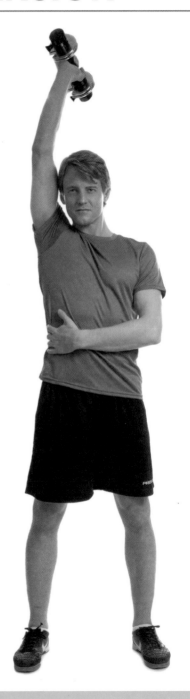

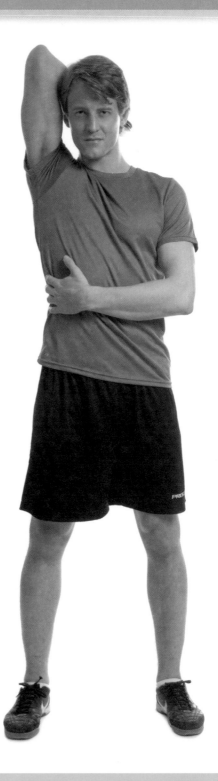

FIND YOUR FORM

- Let the weight pull your arm back slightly to maintain full shoulder flexion.
- Keep your forearm in line with your ear throughout the exercise.
- Place your non-moving hand just under your ribs to stabilize your shoulder.
- Avoid dropping your elbow back or forwards.

CHALLENGE YOURSELF

It (almost) goes without saying that you can increase the level of difficulty and effectiveness of this exercise by increasing the weight of the dumbbells or kettle bells. Make sure you increase the weight gradually over time.

BEST FOR

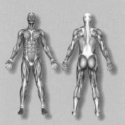

FRONT   BACK

- Hip flexors
- Hip extensors
- Hamstrings
- Quadriceps

ALTERNATING DUMBBELL CURL

1. Stand upright, with your feet planted about shoulder-width apart and your knees very slightly bent. Hold a hand weight or dumbbell in each hand and keep your arms at your sides.

2. In a smooth, controlled movement, bend one arm as you raise the weight toward your shoulder.

3. As you begin to lower your arm, begin to raise the other one, and repeat on the other side.

FIND YOUR FORM

- Keep your knees relaxed throughout the exercise.
- Keep one arm still while the other is moving.
- Move slowly and deliberately, rather than using the weights' momentum to swing them back and forth.
- Avoid arching your back or neck.

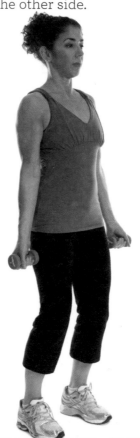

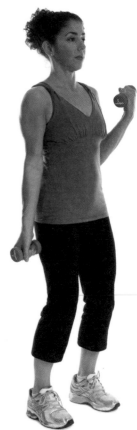

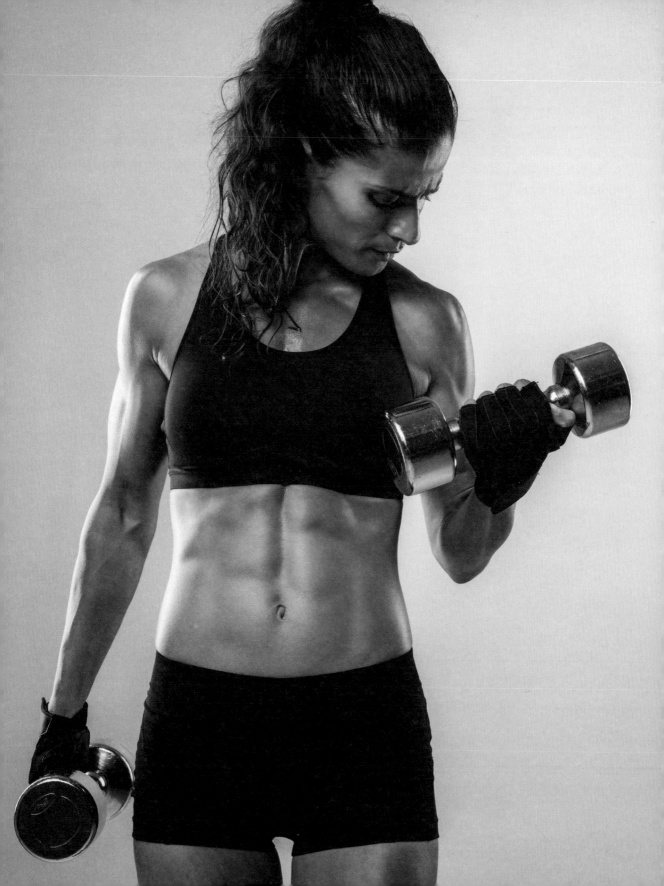

4

TIME ELAPSED

• 2 min

BEST FOR

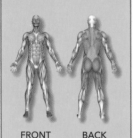

FRONT BACK

• Glutes
• Hamstrings

SINGLE-LEG DEADLIFT

1 Stand on one foot, holding a dumbbell in each hand.

2 Bend forward at the waist, allowing the dumbbells to stretch downward close to your thighs, while keeping a flat back and raising your back leg so that it is in line with your spine.

3 Return to the standing position and repeat, alternating sides with each set.

CHALLENGE YOURSELF

Weighted ankle straps will add a surprising degree of difficulty to this exercise. These straps come in a range of weights, so that you can increase the level of difficulty over time.

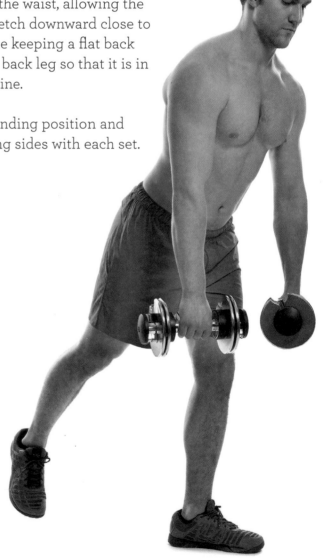

FIND YOUR FORM

- Maintain a full range of motion.
- Keep your knees relaxed throughout the movement.
- Avoid lowering the weights beyond a mild stretch through the hamstrings.
- Avoid rounding your back.
- Move slowly and deliberately or momentum.

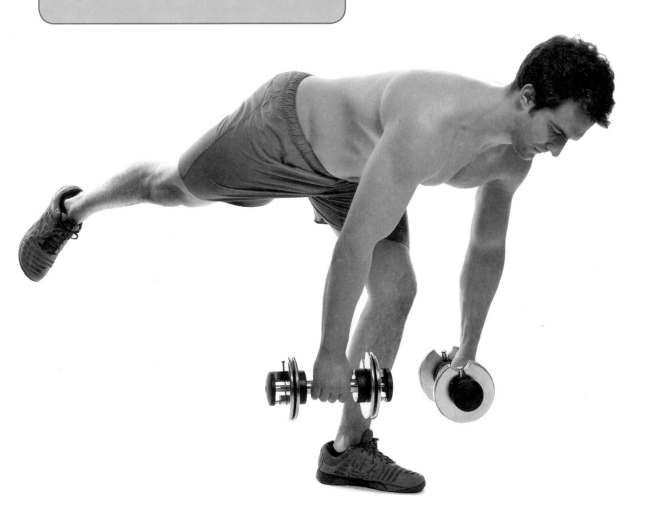

5

TIME ELAPSED

• 2 min, 30 sec

BEST FOR

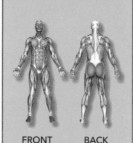

FRONT   BACK

• Glutes
• Thighs

DUMBBELL LUNGE

① Stand with your feet planted about shoulder width apart, your arms at your sides, and a hand weight or dumbbell in each hand.

② Keeping your head up and your back straight, take a big step forward.

③ In one movement as you step forwards, bend your front knee to a 90-degree angle and drop your front thigh until it is parallel to the floor. Your back knee will drop behind you so that you are balancing on the toe of your back foot, creating a straight line from your spine to the back of your knee.

④ Push through your front heel to stand upright, and then return to starting position. Repeat on the other leg.

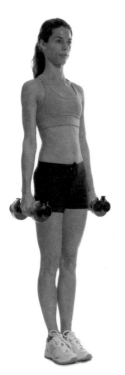

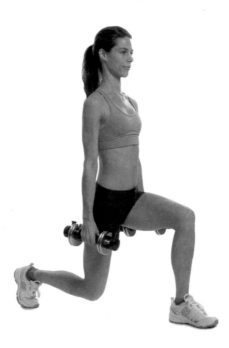

FIND YOUR FORM
• • • • • • • • • • • • • • • • •

• Keep your body facing forwards as you step one leg in front of you.

• Ease into the lunge.

• Make sure that your front knee is facing forwards.

• Avoid turning your body to one side.

• Don't allow your knee to extend past your foot.

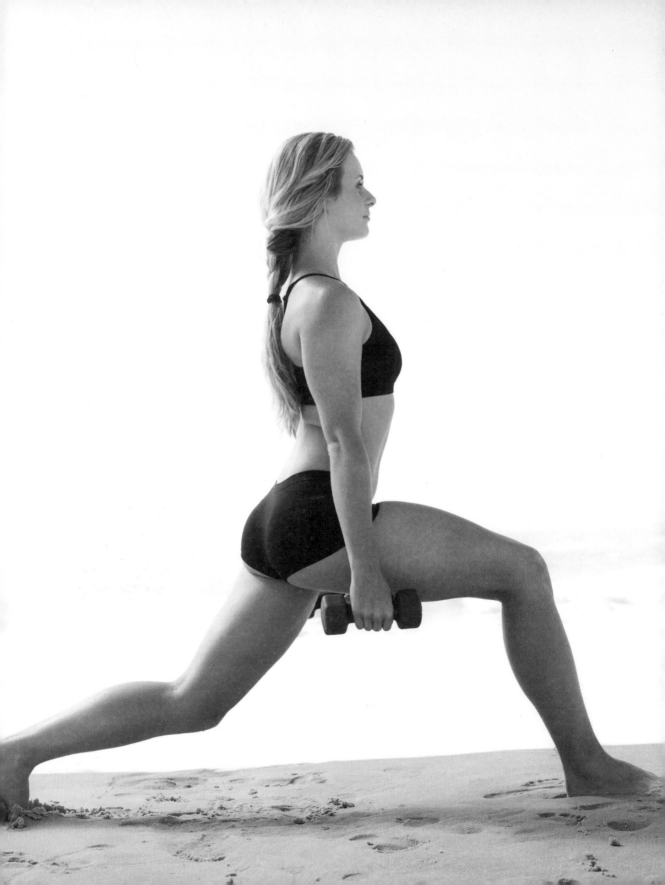

6

TIME ELAPSED

• 3 min

BEST FOR

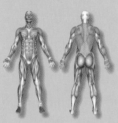

FRONT   BACK

• Shoulders

LATERAL SHOULDER RAISE

1. Holding a dumbbell in each hand, stand with your feet parallel and shoulder width apart and your knees slightly bent. Bend your elbow slightly and face your palms inward.

2. Extend both arms out to the sides to shoulder height.

3. Slowly lower the dumbbells back to the starting position and repeat.

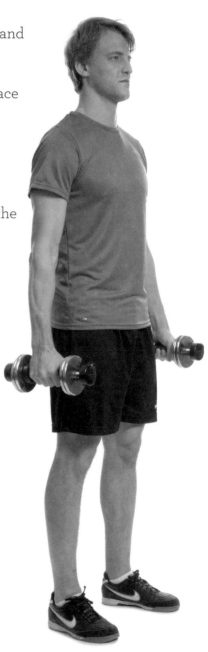

FIND YOUR FORM

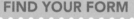

• Keep your elbows in a fixed and slightly bent position throughout the movement.
• Position your elbows directly lateral to your shoulders at the top of the movement.
• Exhale as you lift the dumbbells, and inhale as you lower them.
• Keep your chest elevated.
• Keep your shoulders down.
• Avoid using momentum to lift the dumbbells.

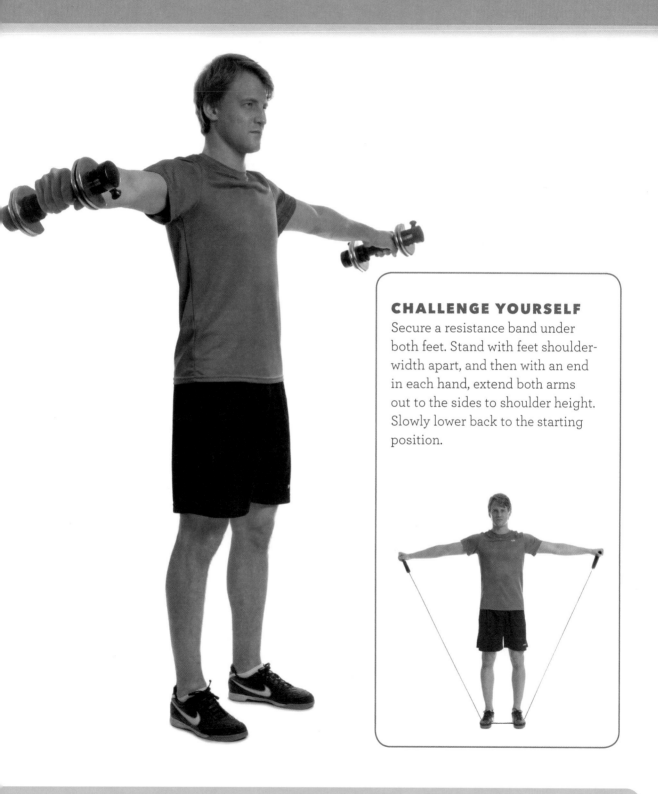

CHALLENGE YOURSELF

Secure a resistance band under both feet. Stand with feet shoulder-width apart, and then with an end in each hand, extend both arms out to the sides to shoulder height. Slowly lower back to the starting position.

TIME ELAPSED

• 3 min, 30 sec

BEST FOR

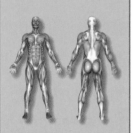

FRONT   BACK

• Shoulders
• Chest

SHOULDER RAISE AND PULL

1 Holding a dumbbell or hand weight in each hand, stand with your legs and feet parallel and shoulder width apart. Bend your knees very slightly and tuck your pelvis slightly forwards, lift your chest and press your shoulders downwards and back.

2 Bring your arms up to a 90-degree angle in front of you.

3 Pull dumbbells to front of shoulder with elbows leading out to sides.

4 Slowly return to starting position and repeat.

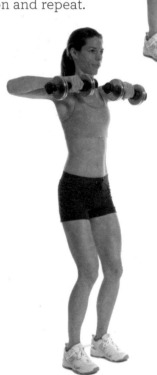

FIND YOUR FORM

• Keep a slight bend in your elbow as you lift upwards to avoid stress on the joints.

• Raising your elbows or the weight higher than your shoulders.

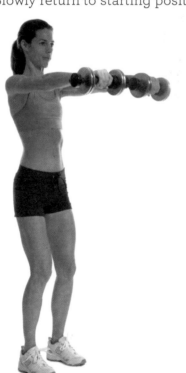

8

TIME ELAPSED

• 4 min

BEST FOR

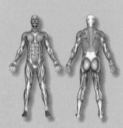

FRONT   BACK

• Shoulders
• Upper Back

DUMBBELL UPRIGHT ROW

1 Stand with your feet parallel and shoulder-width apart, holding a pair of dumbbells in front of your thighs.

2 Bend your elbows to the side as you raise your weights, aiming for shoulder height.

3 Lower the dumbbells to starting position and repeat.

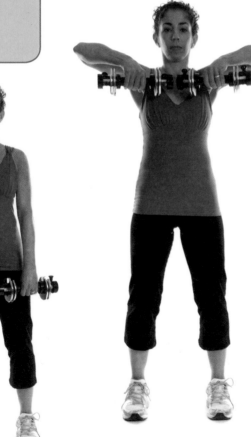

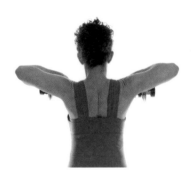

BACK VIEW

FIND YOUR FORM

• Keep your torso stable, your back straight, and your abs engaged.
• Lead with your elbows.
• Avoid swinging your weights; instead, move slowly and with control.
• Avoid arching your back or slump forward.

9

TIME ELAPSED

• 4 min, 30 sec

BEST FOR

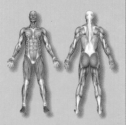

FRONT   BACK

• Gluteal muscles
• Thighs

SUMO SQUAT

1 Stand with your feet apart and turned out, holding a dumbbell between your legs.

2 Keeping your torso upright, bend your knees as you lower into a squat position.

3 Push through your heels as you rise back into an upright position, then repeat.

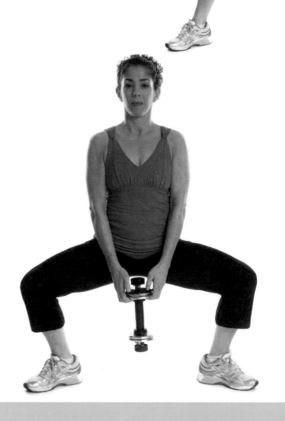

FIND YOUR FORM

• Gaze forward.
• Keep your chest lifted and your shoulders down.
• Engage your core.
• Don't allow your knees to extend past your feet.
• Don't arch your back or slump forward.
• Don't hunch your shoulders.
• Don't twist your torso.

BEST FOR

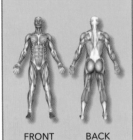

FRONT   BACK

• Calves

DUMBBELL CALF RAISE

1 Stand with your arms at your sides, holding a hand weight or dumbbell in each hand with palms facing inward.
2 Keeping the rest of your body steady, slowly raise your heels off the floor to balance on the balls of your feet.
3 Hold, return to the starting position, and repeat.

FIND YOUR FORM

• Keep your core stable and your back straight.
• Gaze forward.
• Try to balance on the balls of your feet.
• Don't bend your knees.
• Don't rush through the movement.
• Don't arch your back or slump forward.

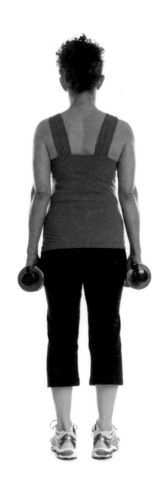
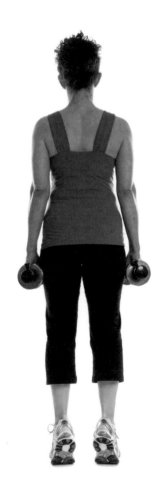

TIME ELAPSED

• 5 min, 30 sec

BEST FOR

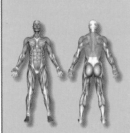

FRONT   BACK

• Thighs
• Shoulders
• Glutes
• Upper back

LUNGE WITH DUMBBELL UPRIGHT ROW

① Stand tall with your legs spaced widely apart holding a pair of dumbbells at arms' length. Step one leg forward and the other back.

② Bend your front knee until your front thigh is parallel to the floor and you can feel the muscles of your rear thigh working. As you bend, simultaneously raise the dumbbells, with your elbows leading, until they are level with your shoulders.

③ Push through your front heel to stand back up into the starting position. Repeat.

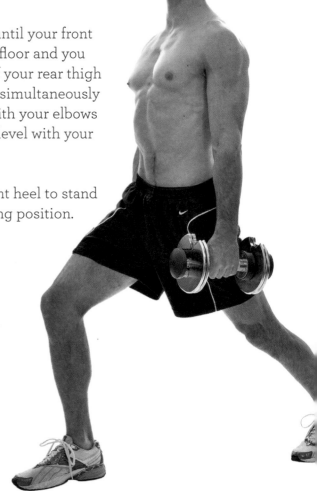

FIND YOUR FORM

• Use your elbows to lead the upright row.
• Avoid hyperextending your knees past your toes.

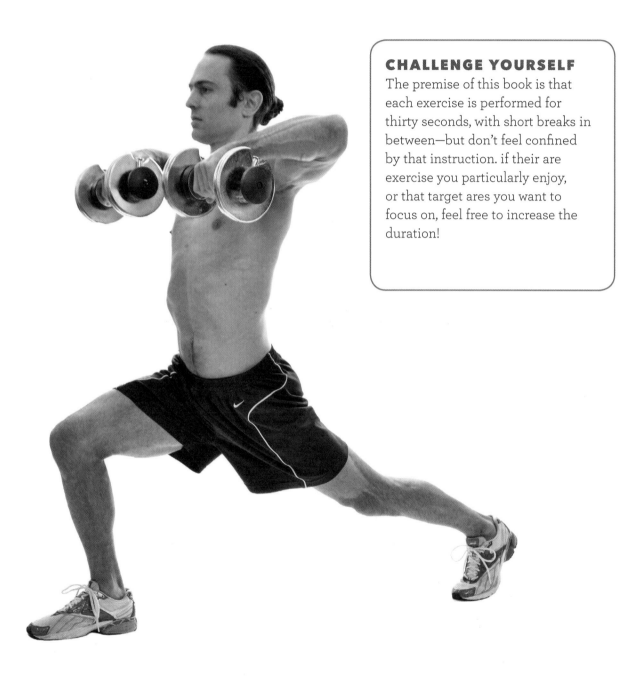

CHALLENGE YOURSELF
The premise of this book is that each exercise is performed for thirty seconds, with short breaks in between—but don't feel confined by that instruction. if their are exercise you particularly enjoy, or that target ares you want to focus on, feel free to increase the duration!

12

BEST FOR

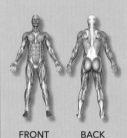

FRONT   BACK

• Shoulders
• Upper Back

SEATED ALTERNATING DUMBBELL PRESS

1 Sit on a Swiss ball in a well-balanced, neutral position, with your hips directly over the center of the ball, grasping a dumbbell in each hand. Hold one to each side of your shoulders with your elbows below your wrists.

2 Press one arm upward to full lockout, and then lower down the same pathway.

3 Repeat on the other arm, and then continue to alternate sides.

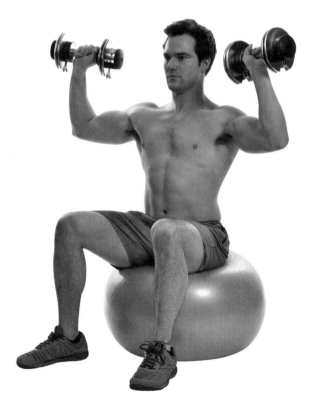

FIND YOUR FORM

- Keep your movements slow and controlled.
- Pause at the top of the movement, and then lower to just above the start position, keeping tension on the muscles until the set is complete.
- Keep your elbows rigid without locking them at the top of the movement.
- Keep your torso stabilized.
- Avoid lowering too far outside your shoulders.
- Avoid tensing your neck.
- Avoid wiggling or squirming in an effort to press the weights upward.

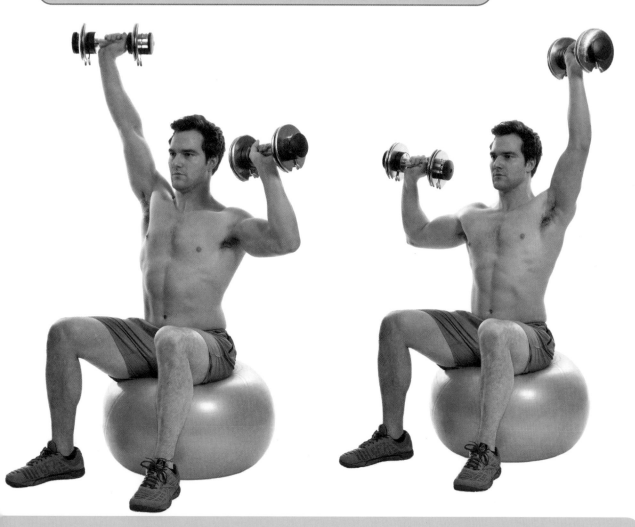

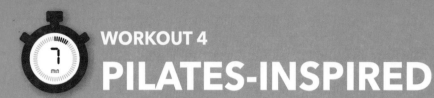

1 Spine Twist

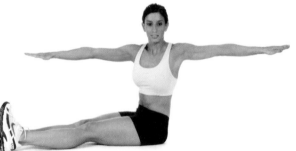

2 Tiny Steps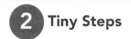

3 Pilates X

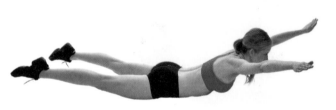

4 Double-Leg Abdominal Press

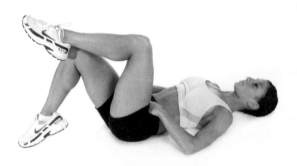

5 Leg Raise

6 Abdominal Kick

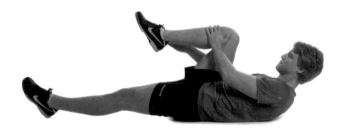

These Pilates-inspired exercises are a good way to focus on strengthening your core muscles while still utilizing your whole body. These exercises are weight-free, primarily relying on body weight and flexibility. If you want to tone your body, improve your flexibility, and keep your joints and muscles relaxed and limber, this is a good place to start.

7 Abdominal Hip Lift

8 Bridge

9 Single-Leg Glute Bridge

10 Front Plank

11 Single-Leg Circles

12 Scissors

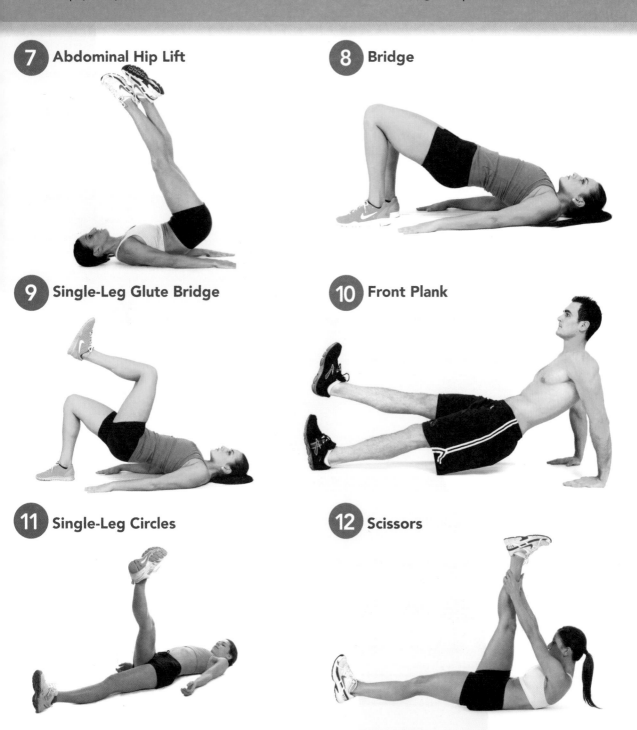

BEST FOR

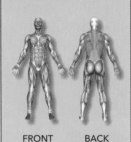

FRONT   BACK

• Back

SPINE TWIST

① Sit on the floor, with your back straight. Extend your legs in front of you, slightly more than hip-width apart.

② Lift yourself as tall as you can from the base of your spine. Ground your hips into the floor.

③ Lift up and out of your hips as you pull in your lower abdominals. Twist from your waist to the left, keeping your hips squared and grounded.

④ Slowly return to the center.

⑤ Lift up and out of your hips again, twisting in the other direction.

⑥ Return to the center. Repeat three times in each direction.

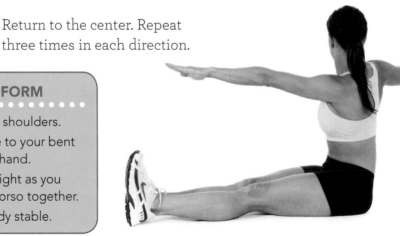

FIND YOUR FORM

• Relax your neck and shoulders.
• Apply even pressure to your bent leg with your active hand.
• Keep your torso upright as you pull your knee and torso together.
• Keep your lower body stable.

2

TIME ELAPSED

• 1 min

BEST FOR

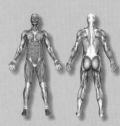

FRONT   BACK

• Abdominals
• Thighs

TINY STEPS

1. Lie on your back with your knees bent and feet flat on the floor.

2. Place your hands on your hip bones to feel if you are moving your hips from side to side.

3. Raise your right knee to your chest while pulling your navel toward your spine. Hold the position at the top.

4. As you continue to pull your navel toward your spine, lower your right leg onto the floor while controlling any movement in your hips.

5. Alternate legs to complete the full movement. Repeat six to eight times.

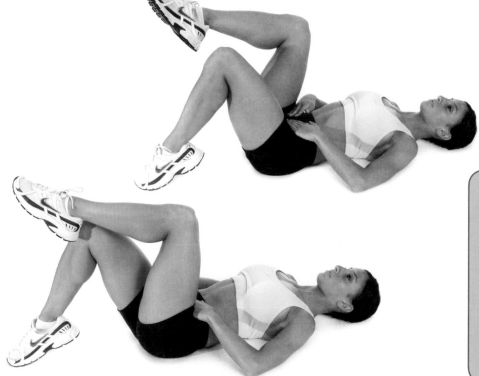

FIND YOUR FORM

• Pull your navel in toward your spine throughout the exercise.
• Avoid allowing your hips to move back and forth while legs are mobilized.

3

TIME ELAPSED

• 1 min, 30 sec

BEST FOR

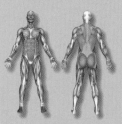

FRONT   BACK

• Hip flexors
• Hip extensors
• Hamstrings
• Quadriceps

PILATES X

1 Lie on your stomach with both your legs and arms fully extended forming an X.

2 Inhale as you simultaneously lift your legs and arms off the floor, tightening your abdominal muscles as you lift.

3 Exhale, draw your legs together, and bend your elbows toward your waist.

4 Repeat for 10 to 12 repetitions.

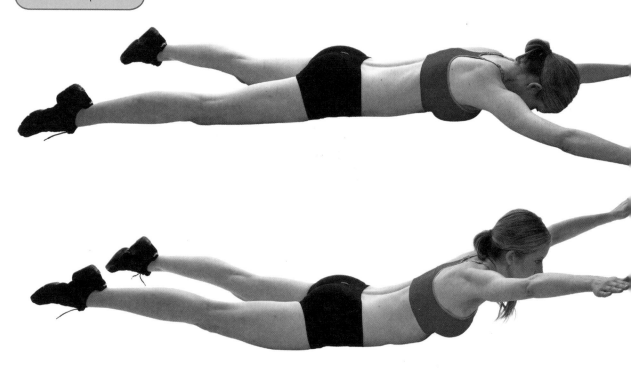

FIND YOUR FORM

- Extend your arms and legs fully.
- Breathe evenly.
- Move slowly and deliberately. Avoid allowing your shoulders to lift toward your ears.

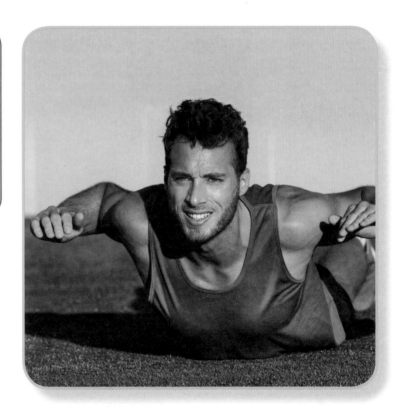

CHALLENGE YOURSELF

The addition of weights will exponentially increase the effectiveness if this exercise—it is already challenging, so there is no need to use heavy weights in the first instance. As with any exercise that involves the use of weights, you can choose whether to use dumbbells, kettle bells, or inanimate household objects. You can also wear weighted ankle straps. Over time you can increase the level of difficulty and effectiveness of this exercise by increasing the weight. Make sure you increase the weight very gradually.

TIME ELAPSED

• 2 min

BEST FOR

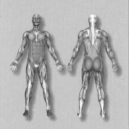

FRONT   BACK

• Core
• Abdominals
• Upper arms

DOUBLE-LEG ABDOMINAL PRESS

1 Lie on your back with your knees and feet lifted in tabletop position, your thighs making a 90-degree angle with your upper body. Place your hands on the front of your knees, your fingers facing upward, one palm on each leg.

2 Flex your feet and, keeping your elbows bent and pulled into your sides, press your hands into your knees. Create resistance by pushing back against your hands with your knees.

FIND YOUR FORM

• Keep your elbows pulled in toward your sides.
• Relax your shoulders and neck.
• Flex your feet and press your knees together.
• Tuck your tailbone up toward the ceiling.
• Breathe evenly while performing the exercise.

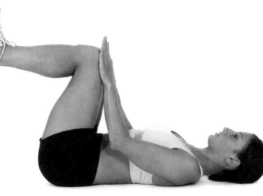

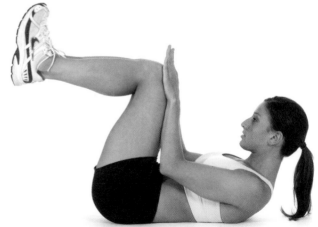

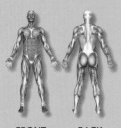
LEG RAISE

① Lie on your back with your arms along your sides. Extend your legs and lift them off the floor, angled away from your body.

② Raise your legs until they are perpendicular to the floor.

③ Lower your legs so that your feet are just above the floor, and then raise them again, performing two sets of 20.

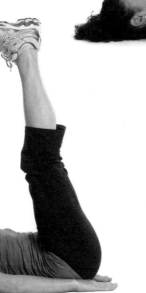

FIND YOUR FORM

• Keep your upper body braced.
• Use your abs to drive the movement.
• Move your legs together, as if they were a single leg.
• Keep your arms on the floor.
• Avoid relying on momentum as you lift and lower your legs.
• Avoid using your lower back to drive the movement.
• Avoid bending your legs.

BEST FOR

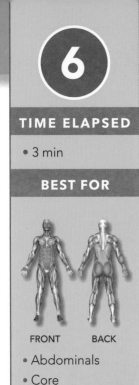

FRONT   BACK

• Abdominals
• Core

ABDOMINAL KICK

1 Pull your right knee towards your chest and straighten your left leg, raising it about 45 degrees from the floor.

2 Place your right hand on your right ankle and your left hand on your right knee (this maintains proper alignment of leg).

3 Switch your legs two times, switching your hand placement simultaneously.

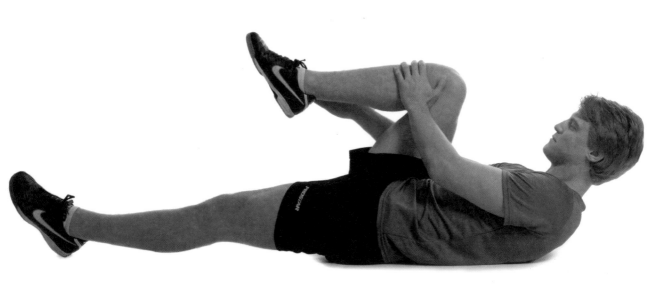

FIND YOUR FORM

• Place your outside hand on the ankle of your bent leg and your inside hand on your bent knee.

• Keep your chest lifted.

• Avoid allowing your lower back to rise up off the floor; use your abdominals to stabilize your core while switching legs.

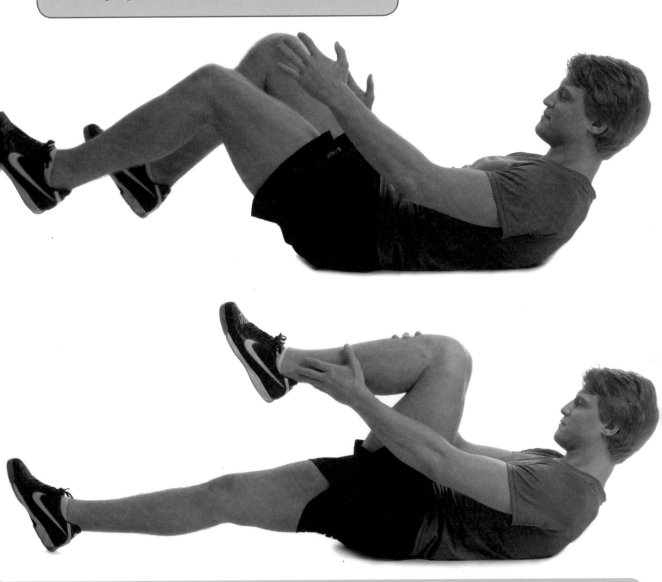

TIME ELAPSED

• 3 min, 30 sec

BEST FOR

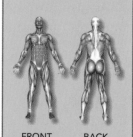

FRONT   BACK

• Abdominals
• Upper arms

ABDOMINAL HIP LIFT

1 Lie down with your legs in the air and crossed at the ankles, knees straight. Place your arms on the floor, straight by your sides.

2 Pinching your legs together and squeezing your buttocks, press into the back of your arms to lift your hips upward.

3 Slowly return your hips to the floor. Repeat 10 times, then switch with the opposite leg crossed in the front.

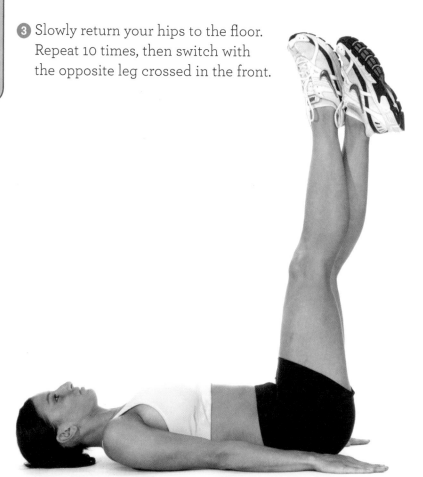

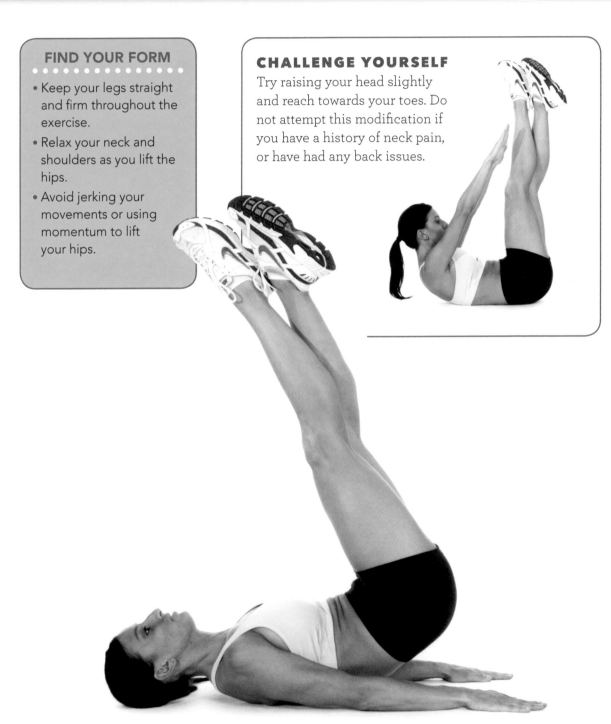

FIND YOUR FORM

- Keep your legs straight and firm throughout the exercise.
- Relax your neck and shoulders as you lift the hips.
- Avoid jerking your movements or using momentum to lift your hips.

CHALLENGE YOURSELF

Try raising your head slightly and reach towards your toes. Do not attempt this modification if you have a history of neck pain, or have had any back issues.

8

TIME ELAPSED

• 4 min

BEST FOR

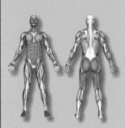

FRONT   BACK

• Glutes
• Hamstrings
• Abdominals

BRIDGE

1 Begin on your back with your legs bent, your feet flat on the ground, and your arms extended on the floor, parallel to your body.

2 Push through your heels while raising your pelvis until your torso is aligned with your thighs. Hold for several seconds, then lower yourself back down. Perform three repetitions.

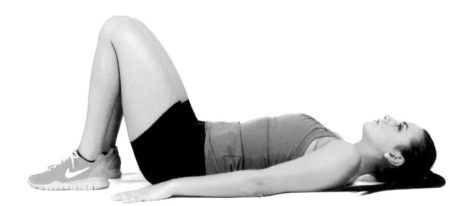

FIND YOUR FORM
• •
• Push through your heels, not your toes.
• Avoid overextending your abdominals past your thighs in the finished position.

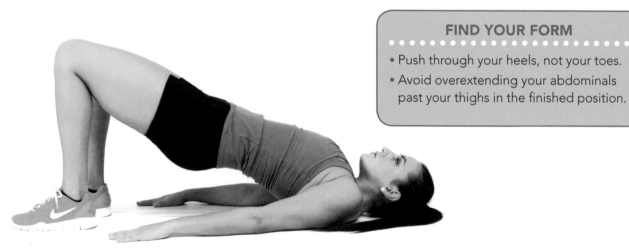

TIME ELAPSED

• 4min, 30 sec

BEST FOR

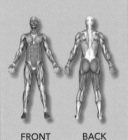

FRONT   BACK

• Glutes
• Hamstrings
• Abdominals

SINGLE-LEG GLUTE BRIDGE

❶ Begin on your back with your legs bent, your feet flat on the ground, and your arms extended along your sides.

❷ Raise your left foot off the floor, keeping your knee bent at a 90-degree angle, until your thigh is perpendicular to your torso.

❸ Push through your right heel while raising your pelvis until your torso is aligned with the planted thigh. Hold for several seconds, repeat, and then switch legs.

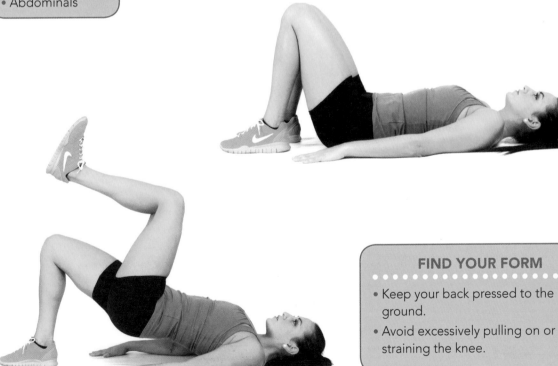

FIND YOUR FORM

• Keep your back pressed to the ground.
• Avoid excessively pulling on or straining the knee.

TIME ELAPSED
• 5 min

BEST FOR

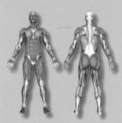

FRONT   BACK

• Shoulders
• Abdominals
• Glutes
• Thighs

FRONT PLANK

1 Sit with your legs extended in front of you and your arms directly behind you, with your fingers pointing straight ahead.

2 Push through your palms and raise your hips and glutes off the ground until your body forms a straight line from the shoulders down.

3 Raise one leg and hold for several seconds, then switch legs.

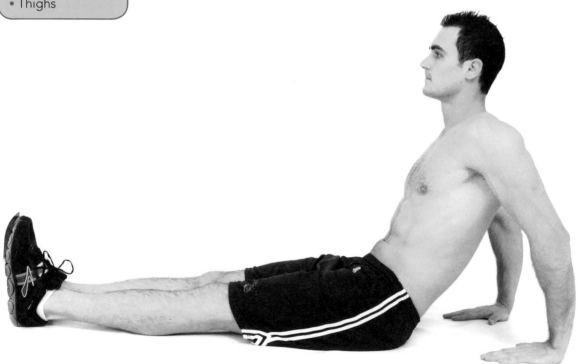

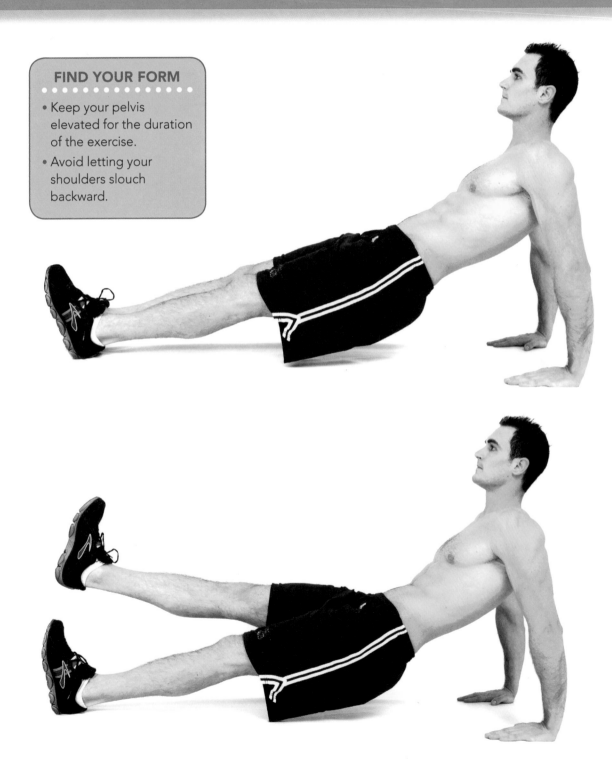

FIND YOUR FORM

• Keep your pelvis elevated for the duration of the exercise.

• Avoid letting your shoulders slouch backward.

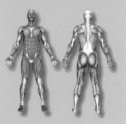

FRONT   BACK

• Abdominals
• Thighs

SINGLE-LEG CIRCLES

1 Lie flat on the floor with both legs and arms extended.

2 Bend your right knee towards your chest, and then straighten your leg up in the air. Anchor the rest of your body to the floor, straightening both knees and pressing your shoulders back and down.

3 Cross your raised leg up and over your body, aiming for your left shoulder. Continue making a circle with the raised leg, returning to the center. Add emphasis to the motion by pausing at the top between repetitions.

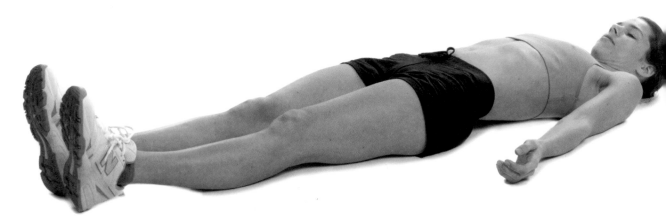

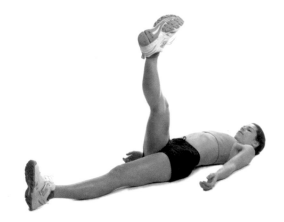

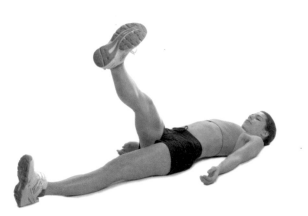

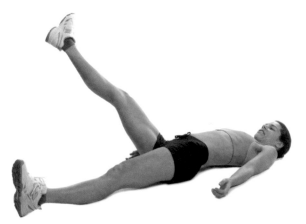

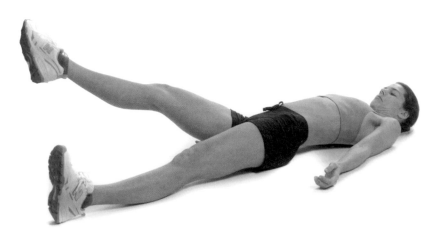

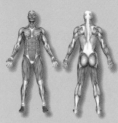
SCISSORS

① Lie on your back with your knees and feet lifted in tabletop position, your thighs making a 90-degree angle with your upper body, and your arms by your sides. Inhale, drawing in your abdominals.

② Reach your legs straight up and lift your head and shoulders off the floor. Hold the position while lengthening your legs.

③ Stretching your right leg away from your body, raise your left leg toward your trunk. Hold your left calf with your hands, pulsing twice while keeping your shoulders down.

④ Switch your legs in the air, reaching for your right leg. Stabilize your pelvis and spine. Repeat sequence six to eight times on each leg.

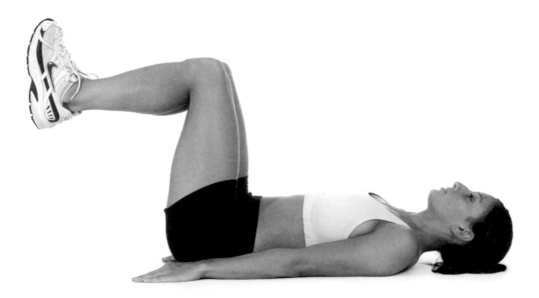

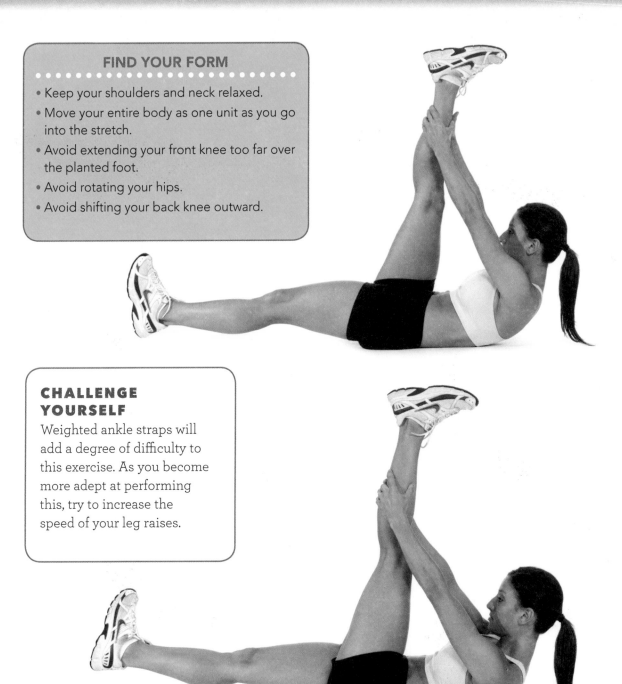

FIND YOUR FORM

- Keep your shoulders and neck relaxed.
- Move your entire body as one unit as you go into the stretch.
- Avoid extending your front knee too far over the planted foot.
- Avoid rotating your hips.
- Avoid shifting your back knee outward.

CHALLENGE YOURSELF

Weighted ankle straps will add a degree of difficulty to this exercise. As you become more adept at performing this, try to increase the speed of your leg raises.

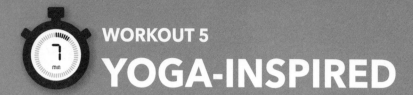

1 High Plank Pose

2 Chaturanga

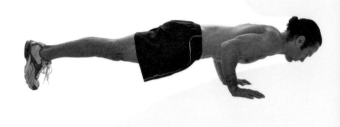

3 Cobra Stretch

4 Upward-Facing Dog

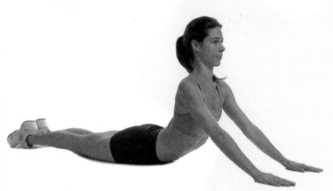

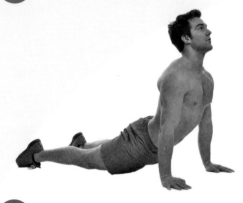

5 Cat-to-Cow

6 Downward-Facing Dog

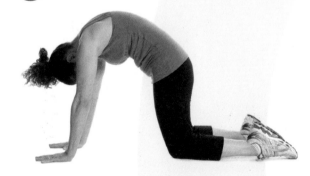

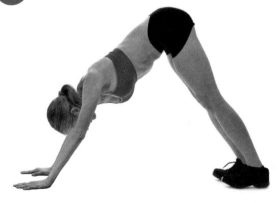

Similar to Pilates, Yoga is intended to strengthen the body, mind, and spirit, with a special focus on flexibility and meditation. These exercises are designed to push the limits of your flexibility, allowing you to increase your effective range of motion while reducing stress and centering yourself emotionally.

7 **Plank Roll-Down**

8 **High Lunge**

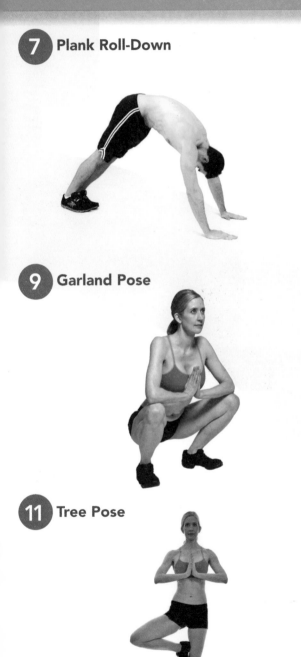

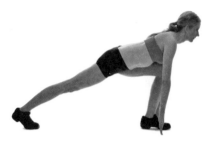

9 **Garland Pose**

10 **Chair Pose**

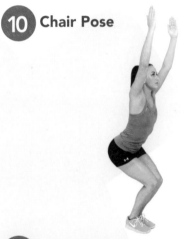

11 **Tree Pose**

12 **Side-Angle Pose**

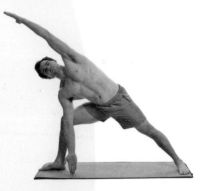

1

BEST FOR

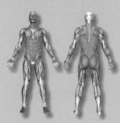

FRONT   BACK

• Abdominals
• Core
• Back

HIGH PLANK POSE

1 Kneel on all fours, facing downward. Your hands should be planted on the floor, shoulder-width apart, and your knees bent at right angles.

2 Straighten your legs and come onto your toes so that your body forms a line. Hold for several seconds.

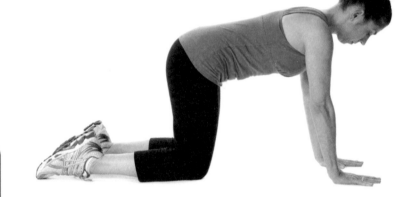

FIND YOUR FORM

• Engage your abs, keeping them pulled in as you hold the position.
• Keep your neck straight and your gaze downward.
• Start by holding for just several seconds, if desired.
• Don't arch your back or allow it to curve forward.

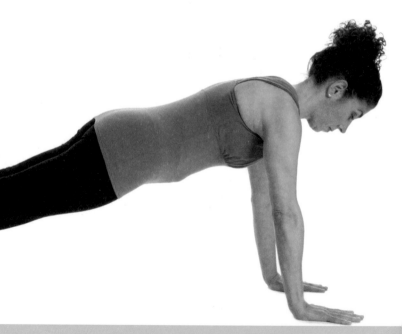

2

TIME ELAPSED

• 1 min

BEST FOR

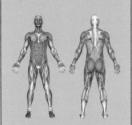

FRONT   BACK

• Triceps
• Shoulders
• Core

CHATURANGA

① Begin in Plank Pose (see opposite).

② Exhale as you lower yourself to the floor, pushing your palms into the ground until your elbows are in line with your shoulders. Keep your body in one straight line and your spine long as you hold for several seconds.

FIND YOUR FORM

• • • • • • • • • • • • • • • • • • •

• Keep your body one long length.
• Spread your fingers wide and ground down through each knuckle.
• Use your breath to get you through holding the pose.
• Avoid rounding your back.
• Avoid dropping your hips lower than your shoulders.

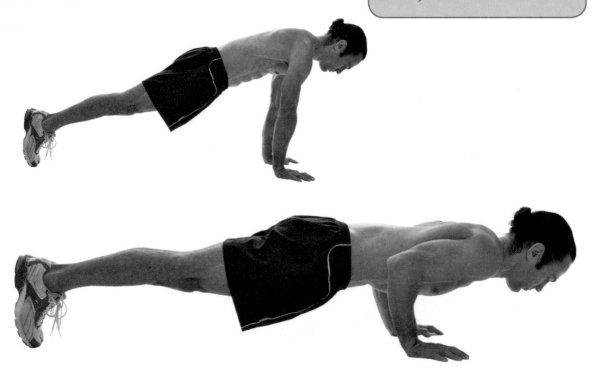

3

TIME ELAPSED

• 1 min, 30 sec

BEST FOR

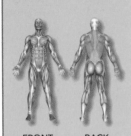

FRONT   BACK

• Back

COBRA STRETCH

① Lie face down with your arms bent, your elbows in, and your palms on the ground.

② Lift your upper body until your arms are at full length. Complete three repetitions of several seconds each.

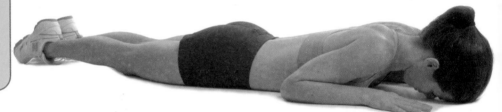

FIND YOUR FORM

• Keep your shoulders and neck relaxed.
• Move your entire body as one unit as you go into the stretch.
• Avoid extending your front knee too far over the planted foot.
• Avoid rotating your hips.
• Avoid shifting your back knee outward.

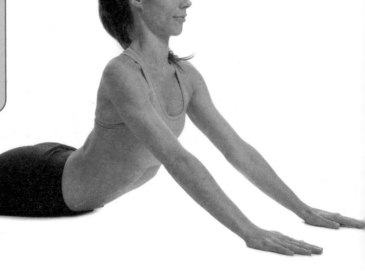

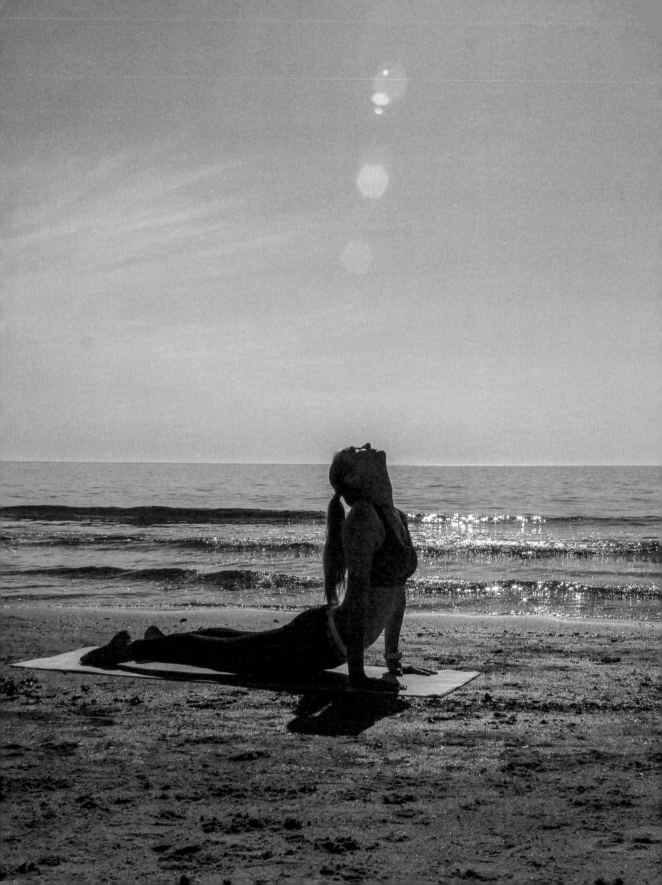

4

TIME ELAPSED

• 2 min

BEST FOR

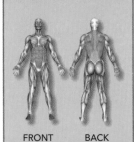

FRONT   BACK

• Back
• Abdominals

UPWARD-FACING DOG

1 Begin in Chaturanga (pp101) , supporting your weight evenly between your hands and feet.

2 Raise your head as you flip the tops of your feet to the floor and straighten your arms with your shoulders above your wrists.

3 Keeping your knees and thighs off the floor, lift your hips and look upward. Hold this position for several seconds.

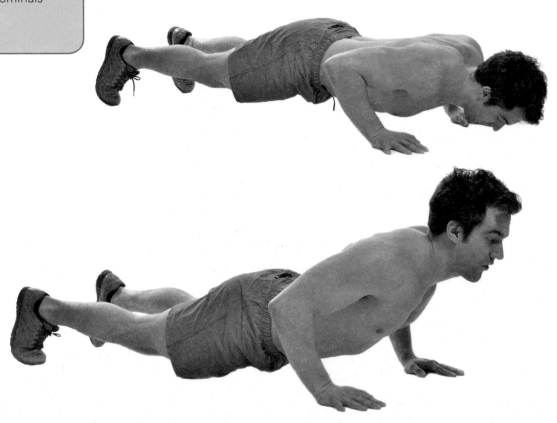

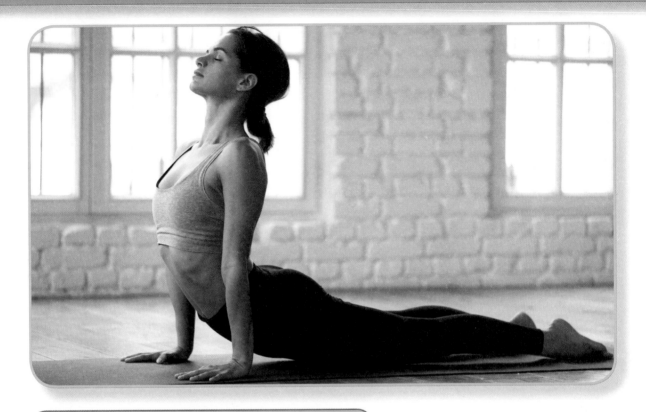

FIND YOUR FORM

- Elongate your legs and arms to create full extension.
- Make sure that your wrists are positioned directly below your shoulders so that you don't exert too much pressure on your lower back.
- Avoid lifting your shoulders up toward your ears.
- Avoid hyperextending your elbows.
- Avoid jutting your rib cage out of your chest.
- Avoid dropping your thighs or knees to the floor.

5

TIME ELAPSED
• 2 min, 30 sec

BEST FOR

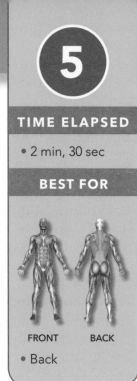

FRONT   BACK

• Back

CAT-TO-COW

① Kneel on all fours, with your back straight.

② Slowly curl your spine, tucking your chin slightly as you take on the position of a stretching cat. Hold for several seconds.

③ Transition to Cow Stretch by releasing the curve of your spine and then moving into a slight arch. Hold for several seconds.

④ Relax and repeat, completing three 30-second repetitions.

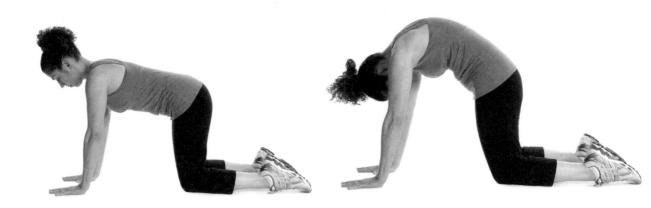

FIND YOUR FORM

• Stretch slowly and with control.
• Keep your hands and feet planted throughout the stretch.
• Lift your chin while your spine is arched.
• Start the movement of your spine in your tailbone.
• Don't curl or arch your back too abruptly.

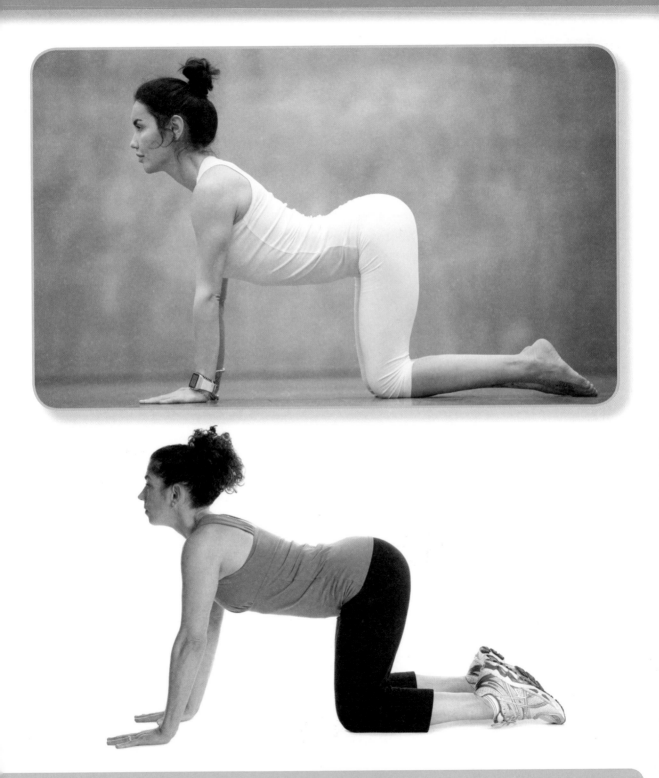

6

TIME ELAPSED

- 3 min

BEST FOR

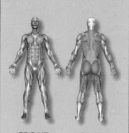

FRONT　　BACK

- Back
- Glutes
- Hamstrings

DOWNWARD-FACING DOG

1 Begin on your hands and knees, with your hands aligned under your shoulders and your knees under your hips.

2 Exhale, and press against the floor, keeping your elbows straight. Lift your sit bones up toward the ceiling and your knees away from the floor. Lengthen your hips away from your ribs to elongate your spine. Hold for several seconds.

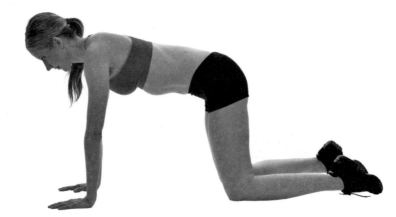

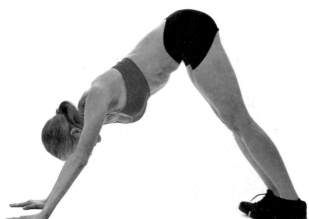

FIND YOUR FORM

- Contract your thigh muscles to further lengthen your spine and keep pressure off your shoulders.
- Press your heels into the floor.
- Avoid sinking your shoulders into your armpits, creating an arch in your back.
- Avoid rounding your spine

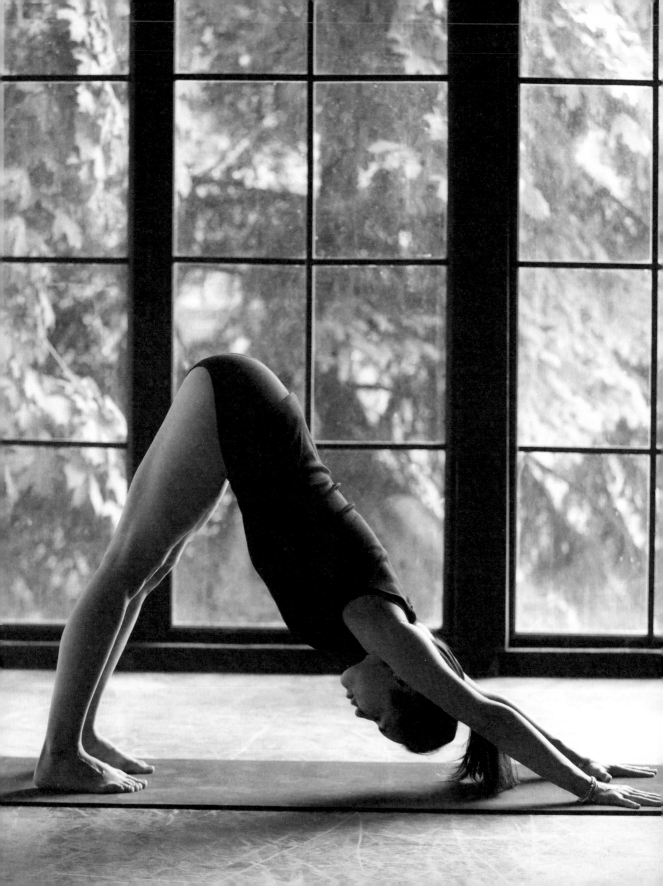

7

TIME ELAPSED

• 3 min, 30 sec

BEST FOR

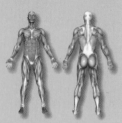

FRONT   BACK

• Biceps
• Triceps
• Abdominals

PLANK ROLL-DOWN

1 From a standing position, bend at the waist, keeping your legs straight as you touch the floor with your hands.

2 Walk your hands away from your feet until you have reached a Plank position on your toes.

3 Once you are in the Plank position, keep your arms straight as you dip your shoulders.

4 Hold for several seconds, then walk your hands back to your feet and return to an upright position. Repeat six times.

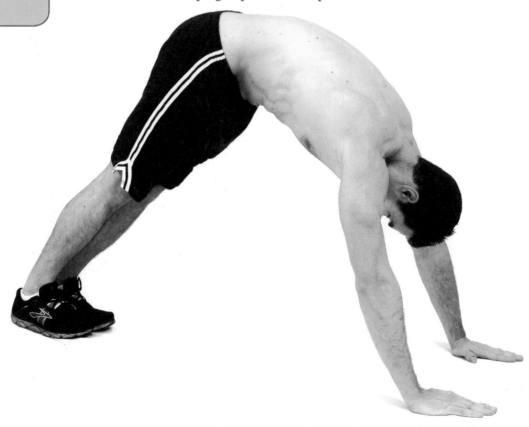

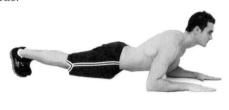

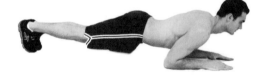

FIND YOUR FORM

- Keep your body straight when in the Plank position.
- Avoid dipping too low, since this can strain the lower back.

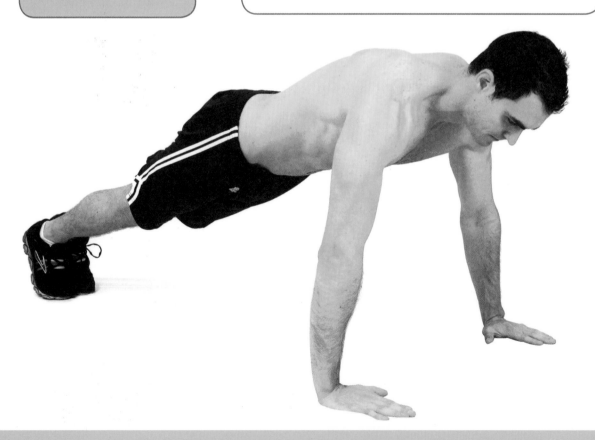

TIME ELAPSED

• 4 min

BEST FOR

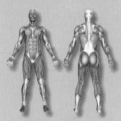

FRONT   BACK

• Outer Thighs
• Hamstrings
• Calves

HIGH LUNGE

1 Stand with your feet together and your arms hanging at your sides.

2 Exhale, and carefully step back with your right leg, keeping it in line with your hips as you step back. The ball of your left foot should be in contact with the floor as you do the motion.

3 Slowly slide your right foot farther back while bending your left knee, stacking it directly above your ankle.

4 Position your palms or fingers on the floor on either side of your left leg, and slowly press your palms or fingers against the floor to enhance the placement of your upper body and your head.

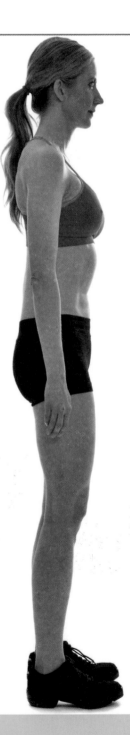

⑤ Lift your head and gaze straight forward while leaning your upper body forward and carefully rolling your shoulders down and backward.

⑥ Press the ball of your right foot gradually into the floor, contract your thigh muscles, and press up to keep your left leg straight. Hold for several seconds.

⑦ Slowly return to the starting position, and then repeat on the other side.

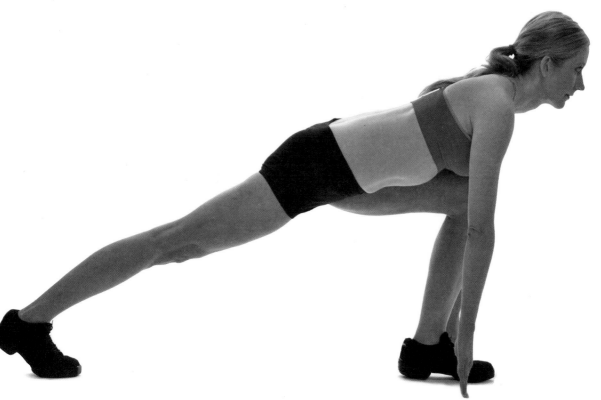

TIME ELAPSED

• 4 min, 30 sec

BEST FOR

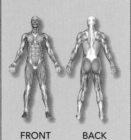

FRONT   BACK

• Glutes
• Thighs

GARLAND POSE

① Stand with your feet shoulder-width apart.

② Planting your feet firmly on the floor, descend to a squat position.

③ Hold the position.

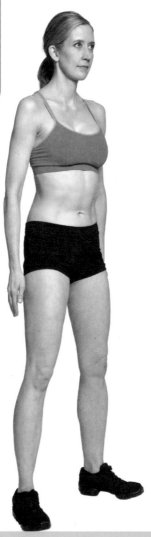

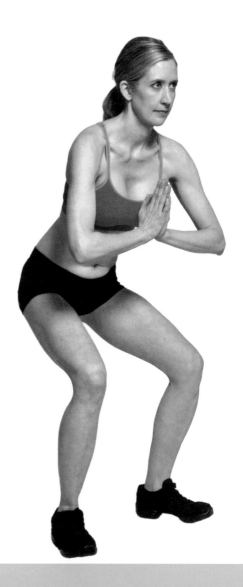

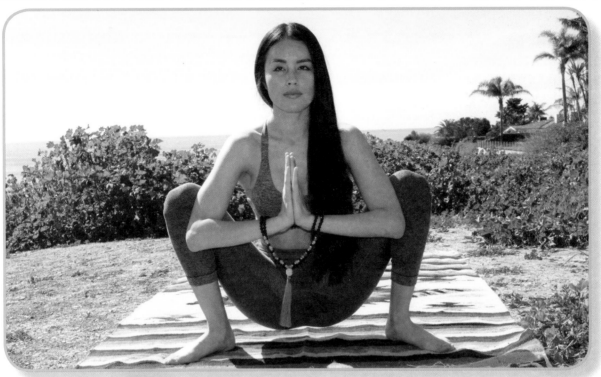

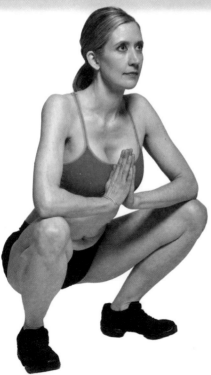

FIND YOUR FORM

- Keep your fleet flat on the floor.
- Keep your spine straight.
- Avoid allowing your knees to hyperextend past your feet.
- Avoid drooping your shoulders or allowing them to move upward toward your ears.

TIME ELAPSED

• 5 min

BEST FOR

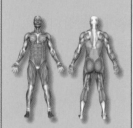

FRONT   BACK

• Thighs
• Lower back
• Calves
• Core

CHAIR POSE

1 Start by standing in an upright position.

2 Raise your arms over your head, bend your knees, and extend your upper body forward to an approximately 45-degree angle.

3 Keep your feet flat and push through your heels.

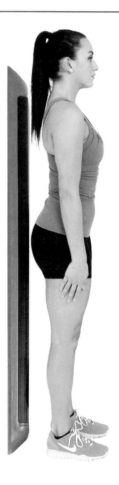

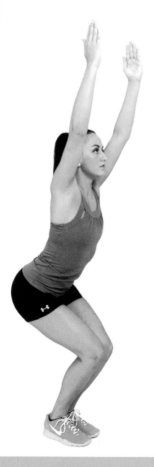

FIND YOUR FORM

• Keep your abdominals contracted throughout the exercise.
• Avoid arching your back excessively.

TIME ELAPSED

- 5 min, 30 sec

BEST FOR

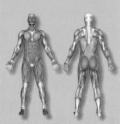

FRONT   BACK

- Gluteal muscles
- Thighs
- Core

TREE POSE

① Stand tall, and then place the sole of your foot against your opposite inner thigh.

② Keep your abdominals braced and bring your hands together in a prayer position. Hold the pose for several seconds, and then repeat on the other leg.

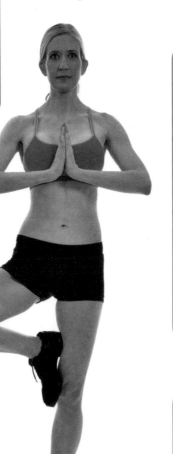

CHALLENGE YOURSELF

Raise your arms upward with your palms facing each other. To make this exercise even more difficult, try doing it with your eyes closed.

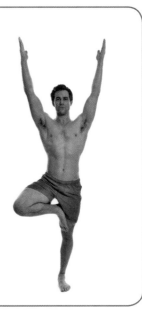

FIND YOUR FORM
• •
- Press your grounded heel into the floor.
- Avoid placing your foot into your kneecap.

TIME ELAPSED

• 6 min

BEST FOR

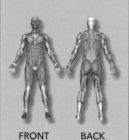

FRONT   BACK

• Core
• Hips
• Thighs
• Back

SIDE-ANGLE POSE

1 Begin in an upright position with your feet spread apart and one foot turned outward while the other faces forward.

2 Extend your arms directly out to your sides with your palms facing downward. Bend your forward knee until it's positioned above your ankle.

3 Bend your torso toward your bent knee, reaching your fingers to the floor as you raise your opposite arm straight toward the ceiling. Take five slow breaths, then return to the standing position and switch sides.

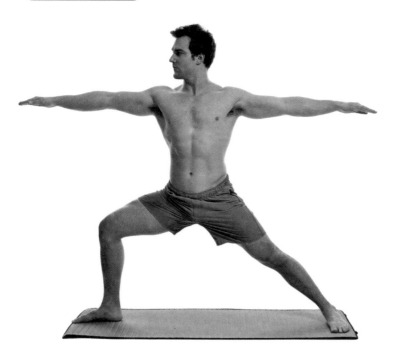

FIND YOUR FORM

• Keep your leading knee tight and aligned with the center of your leading foot, shin and thigh.
• Bend from your hips, not your waist.
• If you feel unsteady, brace your back heel against a wall.
• Avoid twisting your hips.
• Avoid leaning forward—keep your hips and shoulders aligned.

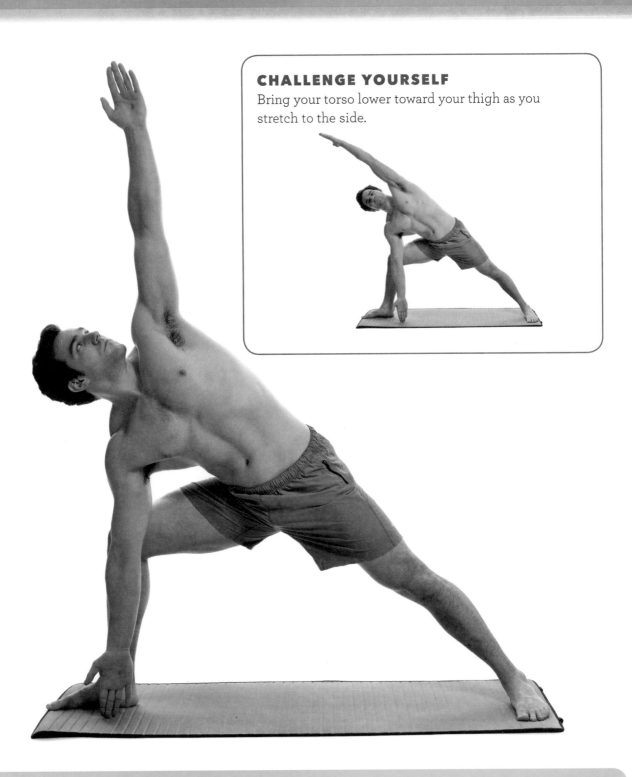

CHALLENGE YOURSELF
Bring your torso lower toward your thigh as you stretch to the side.

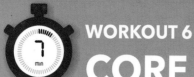
1 Static Sumo Squat

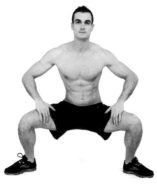

2 Standing Stability

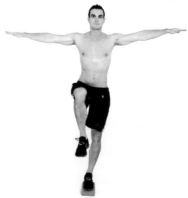

3 Single-Leg Balance

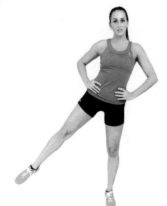

4 Balance Walk

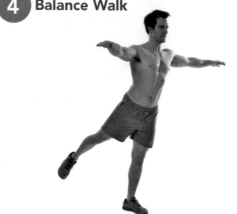

5 Inverted Hamstring

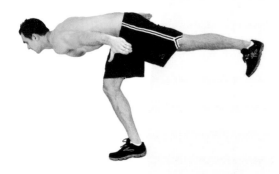

6 Plank Knee Pull-In

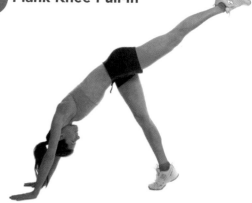

These exercises are intended to help you strengthen your core, improve your sense of balance, and increase your physical stamina. Balance-based exercises are a great way to improve your physical control and core strength, as it takes most of your muscle groups working together to maintain balance in a difficult position.

7 Hand-to-Toe Lift

8 Knee Squat

9 Reverse Lunge

10 Standing Knee Crunch

11 Power Squat

12 Walking Heel-to-Toe

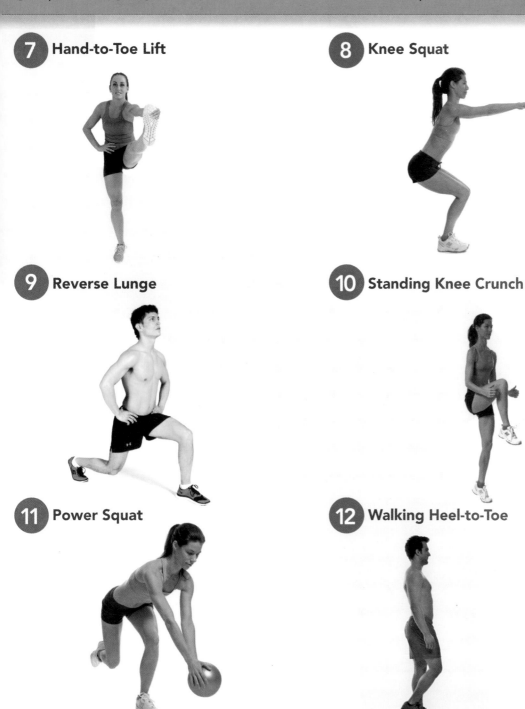

TIME ELAPSED

• 30 sec

BEST FOR

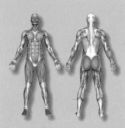

FRONT   BACK

• Thighs
• Gluteal muscles

STATIC SUMO SQUAT

① Stand upright with your feet more than shoulder-width apart.

② Drop down into a deep squat with your hands resting on your inner thighs.

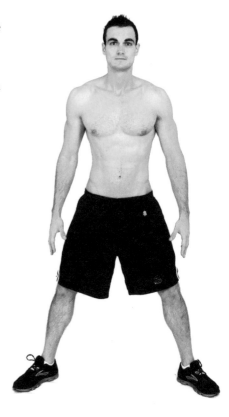

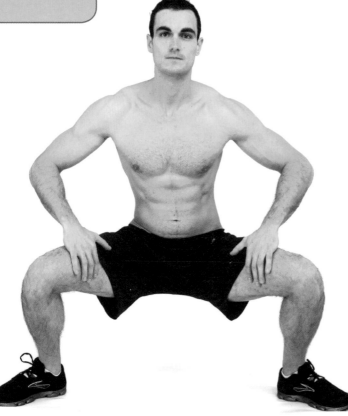

FIND YOUR FORM

• Maintain a neutral spine position.
• Avoid letting your knees extend past your feet.

TIME ELAPSED

• 1 min

BEST FOR

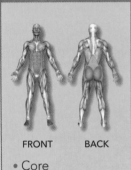

FRONT   BACK

• Core

STANDING STABILITY

1 Begin in a standing position with your left foot on a foam block and your right leg bent at a 90-degree angle.

2 Hold your arms fully extended at 90 degrees to your body, parallel to the ground.

3 Hold for several seconds, repeat, and then switch sides.

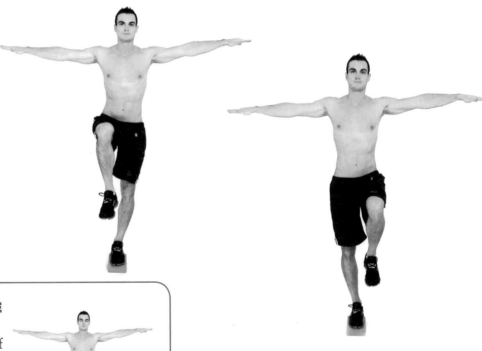

CHALLENGE YOURSELF

To push yourself a little harder, try performing this exercise with you eyes closed.

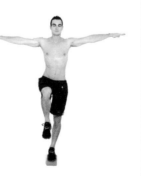

FIND YOUR FORM

• Keep your torso both erect and straight on throughout the exercise.
• Avoid slouching your shoulders.

TIME ELAPSED

• 1 min, 30 sec

BEST FOR

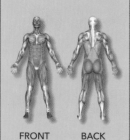

FRONT   BACK

• Core
• Thighs
• Hamstrings

SINGLE-LEG BALANCE

1 Stand with your hands on your hips, and raise your right leg, bent at the knee, directly in front of you at a 90-degree angle. Hold for several seconds.

2 Press your right leg down and forward, though not touching the floor, and hold for several seconds.

3 Finally, press your right leg out to the side, again without touching the floor, and hold for several seconds.

4 Complete the entire sequence three times, then switch legs.

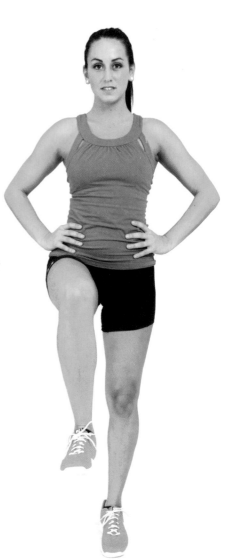

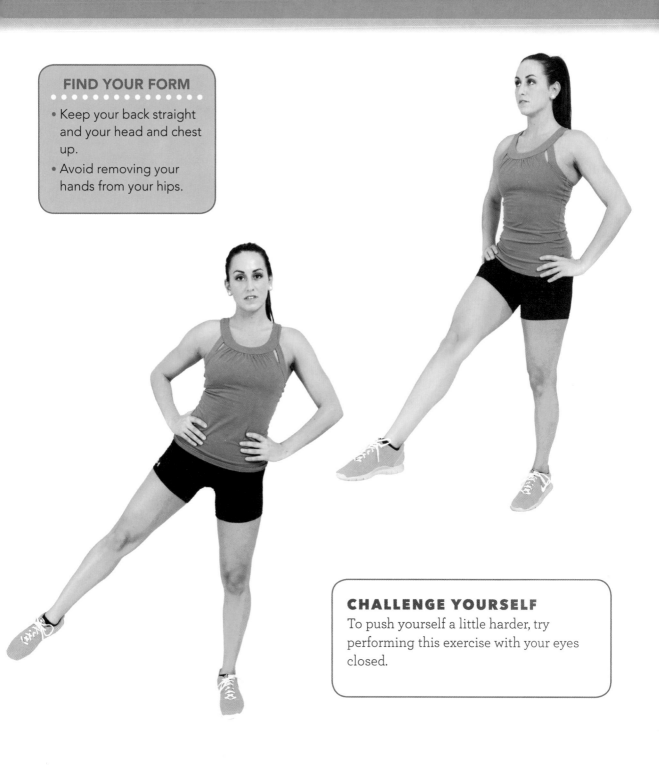

FIND YOUR FORM

- Keep your back straight and your head and chest up.
- Avoid removing your hands from your hips.

CHALLENGE YOURSELF

To push yourself a little harder, try performing this exercise with your eyes closed.

4

TIME ELAPSED

• 2 min

BEST FOR

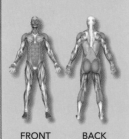

FRONT   BACK

• Calves
• Shoulders
• Core

BALANCE WALK

① Begin by raising your arms out to your sides at shoulder height.

② Choose a target that lies straight ahead and walk in a straight line to get there by putting one foot in front of the other.

③ Lift your back leg as you walk, and then pause for one second before continuing.

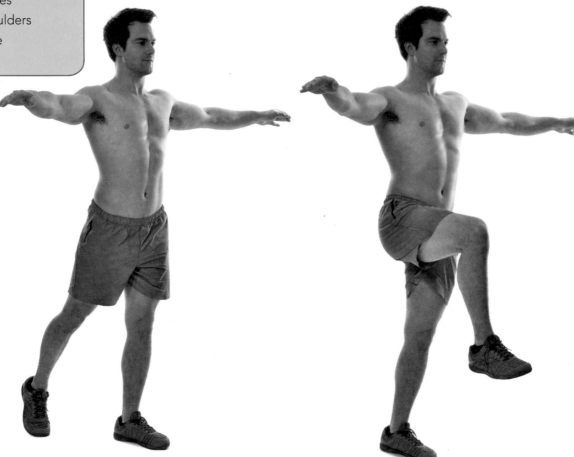

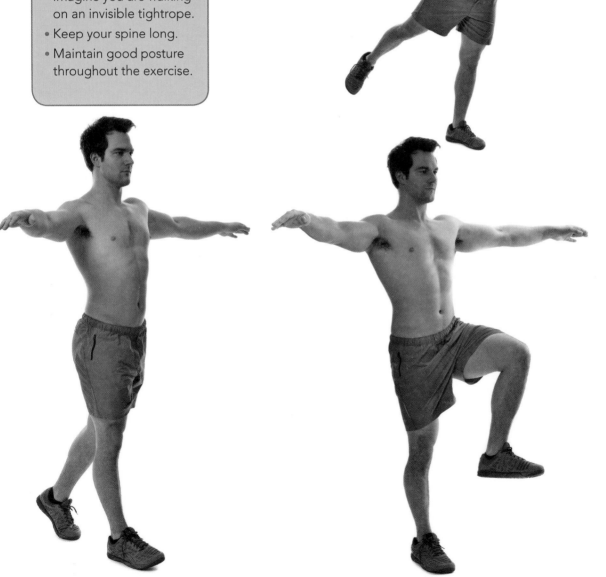

- Avoid slouching or rounding your back.
- Avoid pushing through your toe instead of your heel.
- Imagine you are walking on an invisible tightrope.
- Keep your spine long.
- Maintain good posture throughout the exercise.

5

TIME ELAPSED

• 2 min, 30 sec

BEST FOR

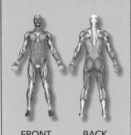

FRONT   BACK

• Hamstrings
• Core
• Glutes

INVERTED HAMSTRING

1 Begin in a standing position, feet shoulder-width apart, with your legs slightly bent and your arms above your head.

2 Bend forward at the waist while simultaneously spreading your arms out to your sides for balance and lifting your left leg behind you, until your torso and leg are roughly parallel to the ground.

3 Hold, then return to starting position and repeat.

FIND YOUR FORM

• Maintain a flat back throughout the exercise.
• Avoid letting your foot touch the ground.

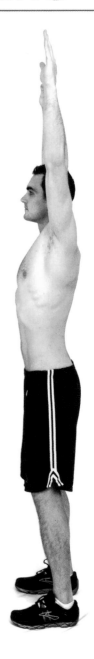

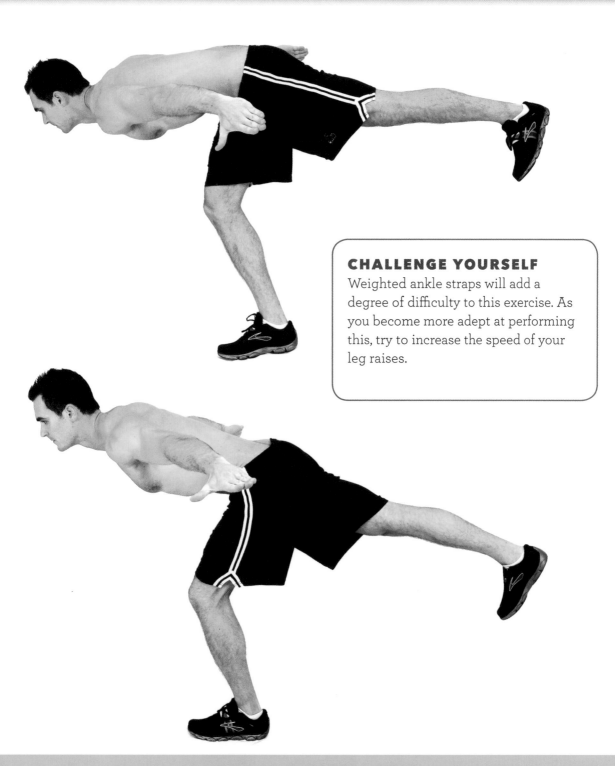

CHALLENGE YOURSELF
Weighted ankle straps will add a degree of difficulty to this exercise. As you become more adept at performing this, try to increase the speed of your leg raises.

6

TIME ELAPSED

• 3 min

BEST FOR

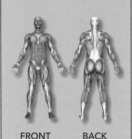

FRONT   BACK

• Abdominals
• Calves
• Shoulders

PLANK KNEE PULL-IN

1 Start in plank position, with your shoulders directly over your hands, your torso straight and your weight distributed evenly between your arms and legs.

2 Draw your left knee into your chest, flexing the foot while rocking your body forwards over your hands. You should come up on the toes of your right foot.

3 Extend your left knee backwards, rocking your body back and shifting your weight unto your heel.

4 With your head in between your hands, straighten your right leg and lift it towards the ceiling. Repeat 10 times on each leg.

FIND YOUR FORM

• • • • • • • • •

• Align your shoulders over your hands.
• Flex your toes inwards during the movement.
• Avoid bending the knee of the supporting leg.

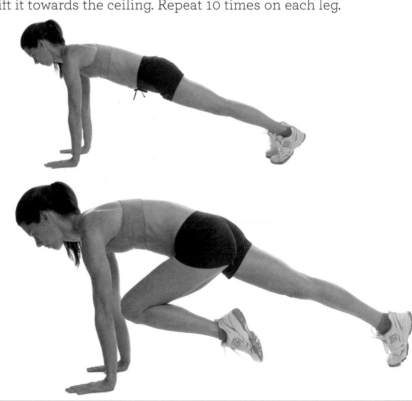

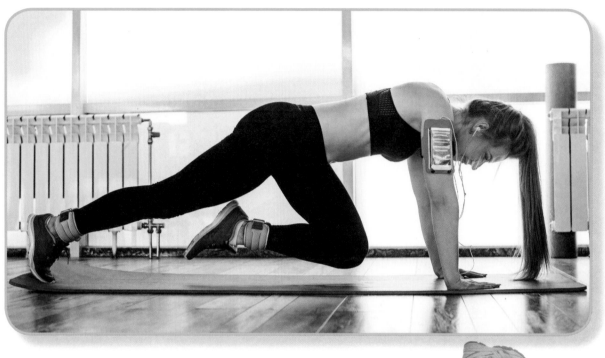

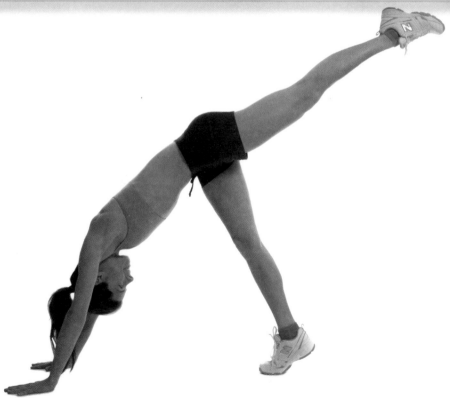

BEST FOR

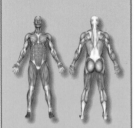

FRONT   BACK

• Abdominals
• Thighs
• Hamstrings

HAND-TO-TOE LIFT

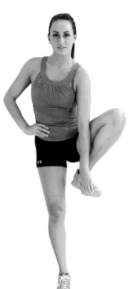

1 Stand with your right hand on your hip and your weight shifted to the right foot.

2 Raise your left knee toward your chest and take hold of your left foot with your left hand.

3 Extend the left leg out in front of you, keeping hold of the toes with your fingers. Maintain the position for several seconds, and then lower the leg. Perform five repetitions per leg.

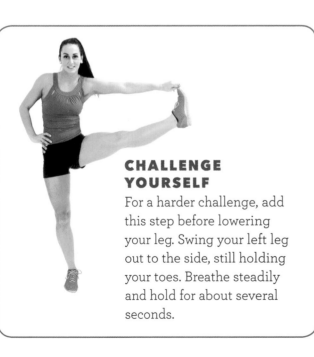

CHALLENGE YOURSELF

For a harder challenge, add this step before lowering your leg. Swing your left leg out to the side, still holding your toes. Breathe steadily and hold for about several seconds.

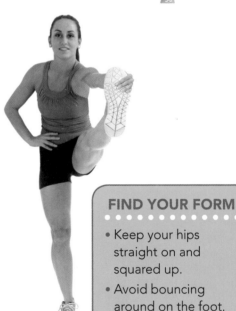

FIND YOUR FORM

• Keep your hips straight on and squared up.
• Avoid bouncing around on the foot.

TIME ELAPSED

• 4 min

BEST FOR

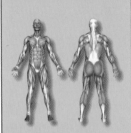

FRONT   BACK

• Gluteal muscles
• Quadriceps
• Hip flexors

KNEE SQUAT

1 Stand with your legs and feet parallel and shoulder-width apart, and your knees bent very slightly. Tuck your pelvis slightly forwards, lift your chest, and press your shoulders down and back.

2 Extend your arms in front of your body for stability, keeping them even with your shoulders. With your feet planted firmly on the floor, curl

3 Draw in your abdominal muscles and bend into a squat Keep your heels planted on the floor and your chest as upright as possible, resisting the urge to bend too far forwards.

4 Exhale, and return to the original position. Repeat five to six times.

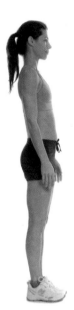

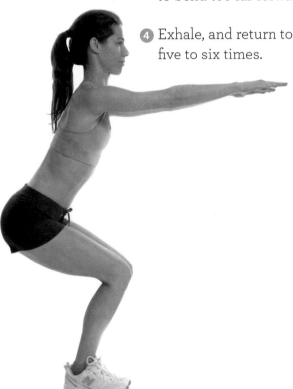

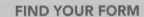

FIND YOUR FORM

• Keep your chest upright.
• Pull your abdominals in towards your spine.
• Curl your toes upwards throughout the movement.
• Imagine pressing into the floor as you rise from the squat, creating your body's own resistance in your leg muscles.
• Avoid allowing your heels to lift off the floor.
• Avoid rising too quickly to the standing position.

TIME ELAPSED

- 4 min, 30 sec

BEST FOR

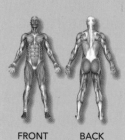

FRONT   BACK

- Glutes
- Thighs

REVERSE LUNGE

1 Stand with your hands on your hips and your feet shoulder-width apart. Take a big step backwards, bending your knees as you do so.

2 When the front thigh is roughly parallel to the ground, push through your front heel to return to the starting position. Perform 15 repetitions per leg.

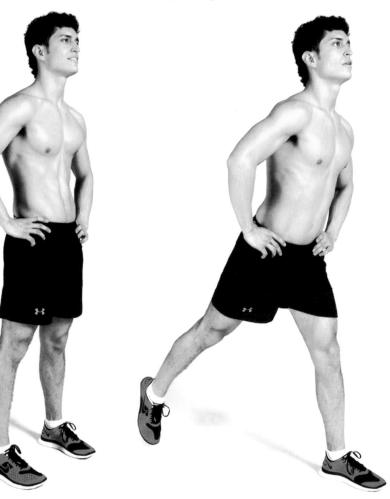

CHALLENGE YOURSELF

More difficult: Hold a pair of dumbbells for increased resistance.

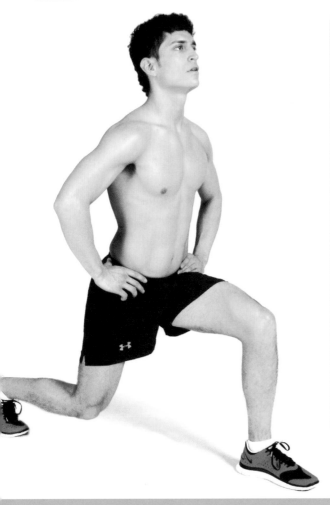

- Keep your shoulders and neck relaxed.
- Move your entire body as one unit as you go into the stretch.
- Avoid extending your front knee too far over the planted foot.
- Avoid rotating your hips.
- Avoid shifting your back knee outward.

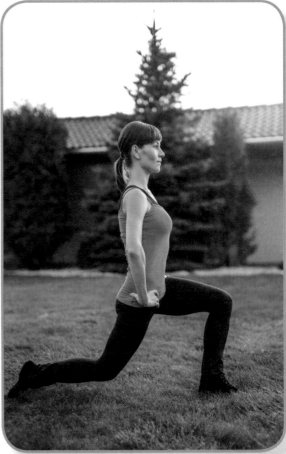

BEST FOR

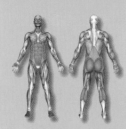

FRONT   BACK

• Calves
• Gluteal muscles
• Core

STANDING KNEE CRUNCH

1. Stand tall with your left leg in front of the right, and extend your hands up toward the ceiling, your arms straight.

2. Shift your weight onto your left foot and raise your right knee to the height of your hips while pulling your elbows down to your sides.

3. Pause at the top of the movement, and then return to the starting position.

4. Switch legs and repeat.

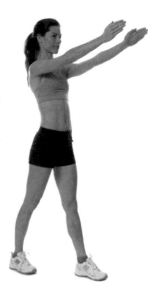

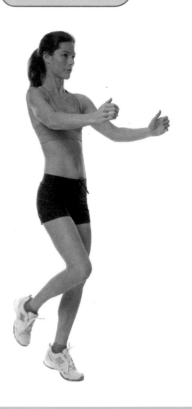

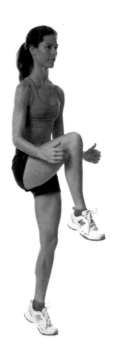

FIND YOUR FORM

• Keep your standing leg straight as you raise up on your toes.
• Relax your shoulders as you pull your arms down for the crunch.
• Flex the toes of your raised leg.
• Avoid tilting forward as you switch legs.

TIME ELAPSED

• 5 min, 30 sec

BEST FOR

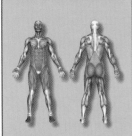

FRONT   BACK

• Glutes
• Thighs
• Core

POWER SQUAT

1. Stand straight, holding a weighted medicine ball in front of your torso.

2. Shift your weight to your left foot, and bend your right knee, lifting your right foot towards your buttocks. Bend your elbows and draw the ball towards the outside of your right ear.

3. Keeping your back straight, bend at your hip and knee. Lower your torso towards your left side bringing the ball towards your left ankle.

4. Press into your left leg and straighten into your knee and torso, returning to the starting position. Repeat 15 times for two sets on each leg.

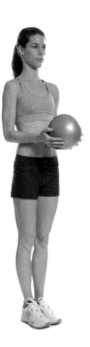

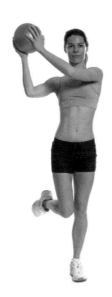
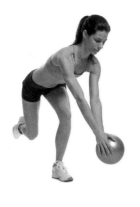

FIND YOUR FORM

• Keep your hips and knees aligned throughout the movement.
• Relax your neck and shoulders
• Move the ball in an arc through the air.
• Avoid allowing your knee to extend beyond your toes as you bend and rotate.
• Avoid moving your foot from its starting position.
• Avoid flexing your spine.

TIME ELAPSED

• 6 min

BEST FOR

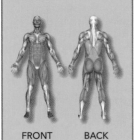

FRONT   BACK

• Calves
• Thighs
• Core

WALKING HEEL-TO-TOE

① Begin standing while positioning the heel of one foot just past the toes of the other, while the two are just barely touching.

② Choose a target that lies straight ahead, and place one foot repeatedly ahead of the other while walking a straight line to get there.

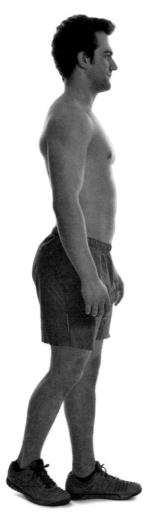

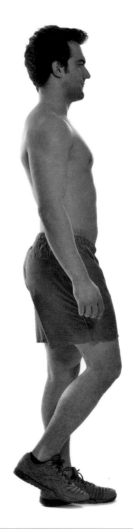

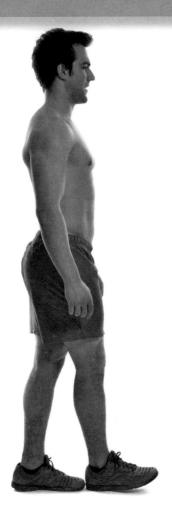

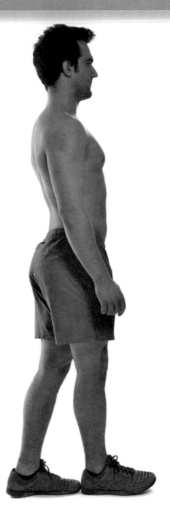

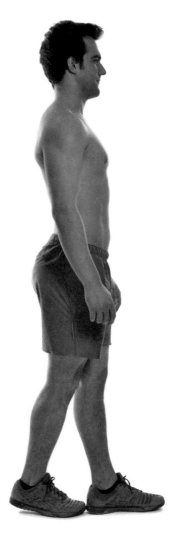

FIND YOUR FORM
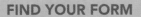
- Keep your spine long.
- Maintain good posture throughout the exercise.
- Avoid slouching or rounding your back.
- Avoid pushing through your toe instead of your heel.

UPPER-BODY/CORE FOCUS

1 **Seated Russian Twist**

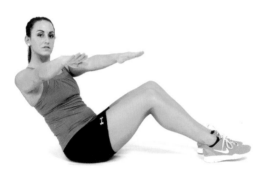

2 **Swimming**

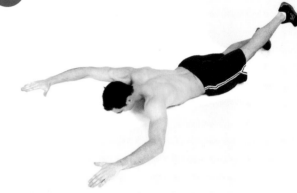

3 **Towel Fly**

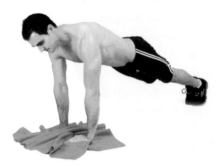

4 **Push-Up**

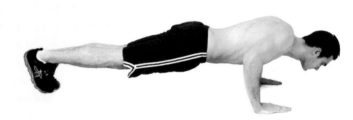

5 **T-Stabilization**

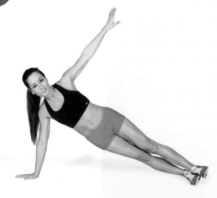

6 **Push-Up Hand Walkover**

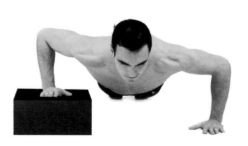

This workout is a great way to strengthen your shoulders, arms, chest, and back while still utilizing your entire body. Exercises like push-ups and t-stabilizations, for instance, utilize a surprising number of muscle groups for support and stabilization.

7 **Plank Leg Extension**

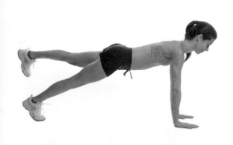

8 **Kettlebell Figure 8**

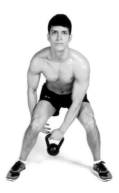

9 **Alternating Kettlebell Row**

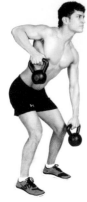

10 **Alternating Kettlebell Press**

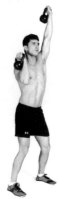

11 **One-Armed Row**

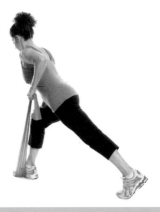

12 **One-Armed Triceps Kickback**

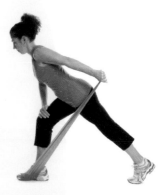

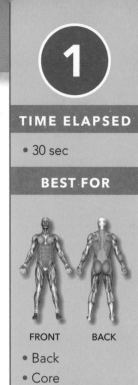
SEATED RUSSIAN TWIST

1 Sit upright with your legs bent and your feet flat on the floor.

2 Extend your arms straight ahead and lean back slightly to activate your core.

3 In a smooth motion, rotate your upper body to the side, and then return to the center.

4 Repeat the rotation on the other side.

5 Return to the center and continue alternating sides.

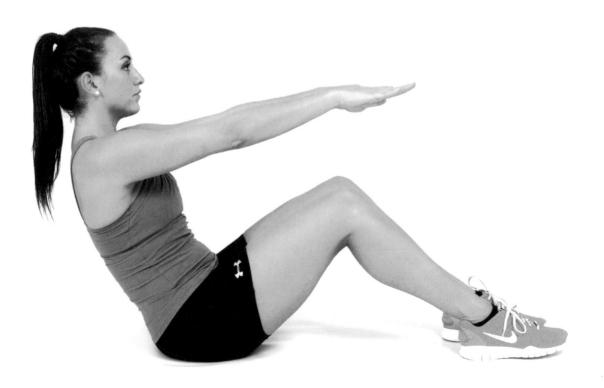

FIND YOUR FORM

- Twist smoothly and with control, keeping your back flat.
- Avoid shifting your feet or knees as you twist.

CHALLENGE YOURSELF

Any exercise can be enhanced by adding the use of weights, you can choose whether to use dumbbells, kettle bells, or inanimate household objects, and you should start with a weight you feel comfortable with. Over time you can increase the level of difficulty and effectiveness of this exercise by increasing the weight. Make sure you increase the weight gradually.

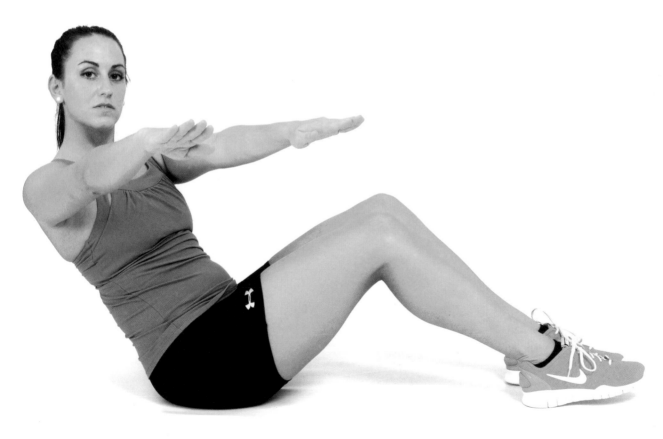

TIME ELAPSED

• 1 min

BEST FOR

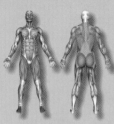

FRONT   BACK

• Back
• Gluteal muscles
• Thighs

SWIMMING

1 Lie on your stomach with your arms stretched out in front of you and your legs stretched out behind.

2 Raise your left arm and right leg off the floor at the same time, along with your head and shoulders, then lower them all back down.

3 Repeat the exercise with your opposite limbs.

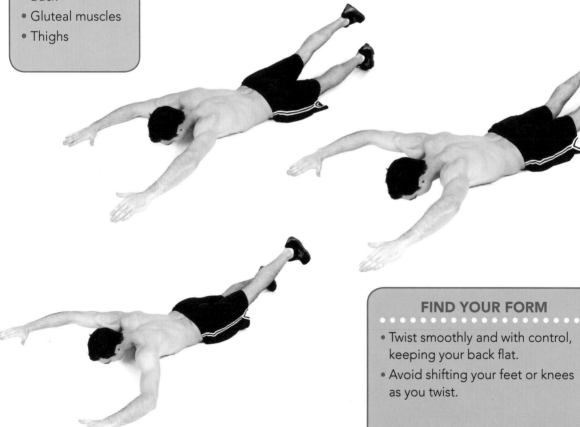

FIND YOUR FORM

• Twist smoothly and with control, keeping your back flat.
• Avoid shifting your feet or knees as you twist.

TIME ELAPSED

• 1 min, 30 sec

BEST FOR

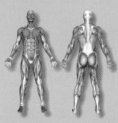

FRONT   BACK

• Shoulders
• Chest
• Triceps

TOWEL FLY

1 Begin in a standard pushup position with a towel on the floor under your chest. Place your hands on the towel, a little more than shoulder-width apart.

2 Keeping your torso still, slide your hands together and then slide them back to the starting position.

3 Repeat.

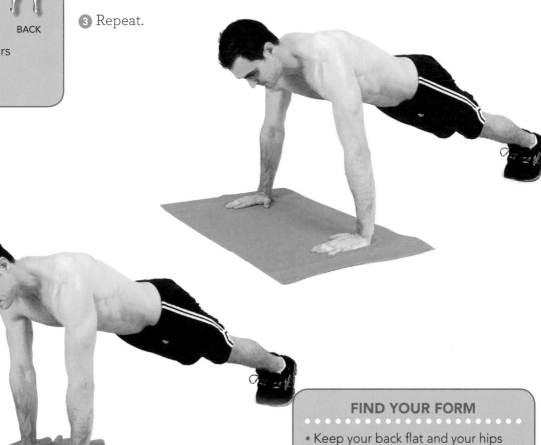

FIND YOUR FORM

• Keep your back flat and your hips raised. Avoid Bending or extending your elbows.

4

TIME ELAPSED

• 2 min

BEST FOR

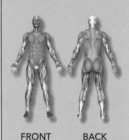

FRONT   BACK

• Chest
• Back
• Shoulders
• Core

PUSH-UP

1 Lie face-down on the ground with your hands planted on the floor shoulder-width apart and your arms fully extended.

2 Lengthen your legs and balance on your toes.

3 Bend your arms until your chest is nearly touching the floor, then push back to full extension.

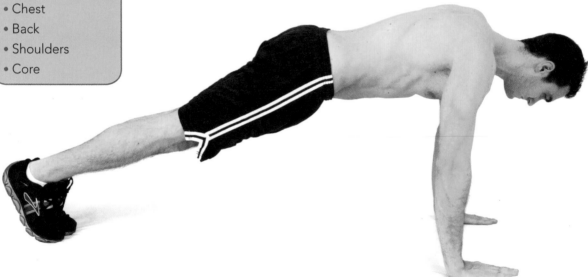

FIND YOUR FORM

• Avoid arching your back.
• Keep your chest directly over your hands.

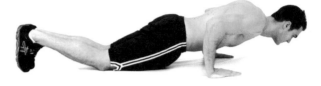

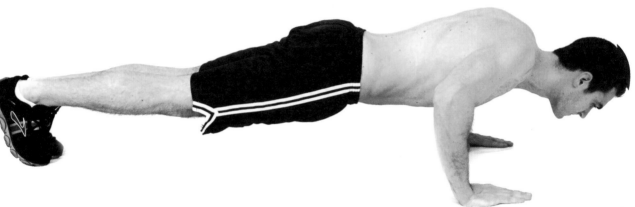

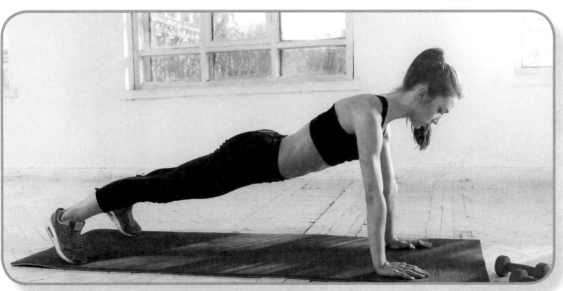

5

TIME ELAPSED

• 2 min, 30 sec

BEST FOR

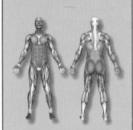

FRONT   BACK

• Core
• Abdominals
• Lower Back

T-STABILIZATION

1. Start in the finished push-up position, with your arms extended to full lockout and your palms facing forwards, supporting yourself on your toes.

2. While keeping your body in one straight line, turn your left hip skywards, allowing your left foot to rest on the right.

3. Raise your right arm laterally across your body until it points to the ceiling. Hold this position for several seconds.

4. Return to the starting position and repeat with the other side.

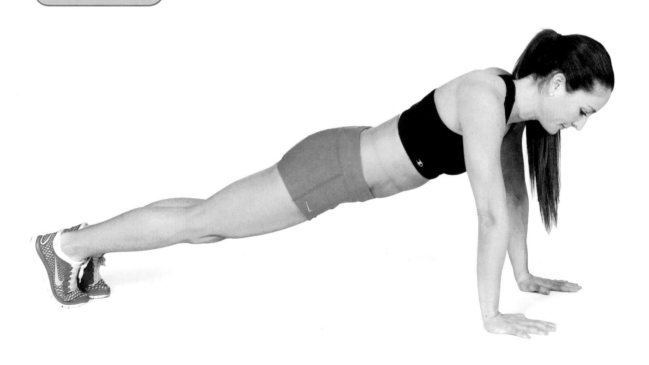

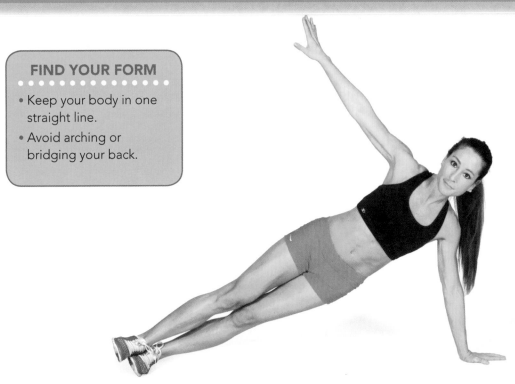

FIND YOUR FORM
· Keep your body in one straight line.
· Avoid arching or bridging your back.

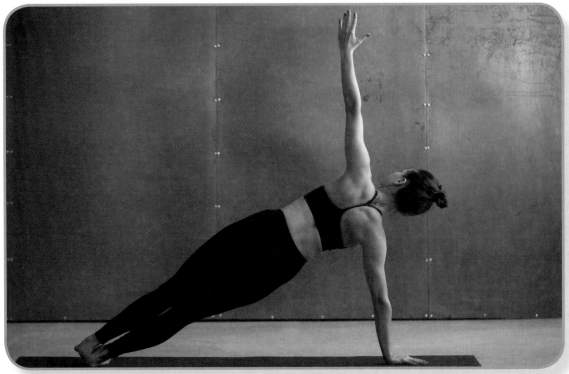

BEST FOR

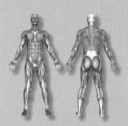

FRONT	BACK

• Chest
• Upper Back
• Shoulders
• Triceps

PUSH-UP HAND WALKOVER

1 Begin in a raised push-up position with your hands close together on a solid block.

2 Move your left hand from the block and place it on the floor as far to the left as is comfortable. Lower yourself to the ground as you would in a normal push-up.

3 As you push back up, move your left arm back to the block and repeat the movement with your right hand out to the side.

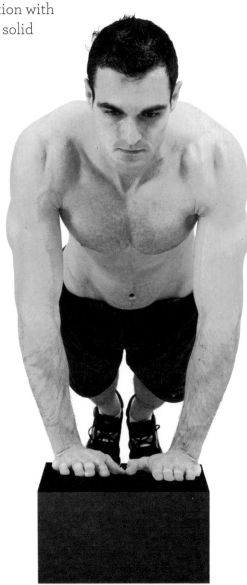

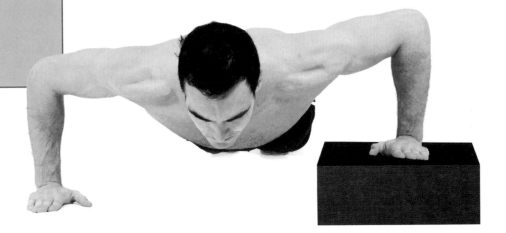

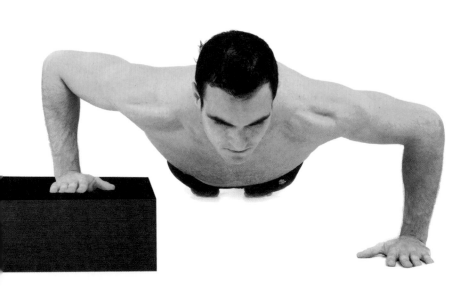

TIME ELAPSED

• 3 min, 30 sec

BEST FOR

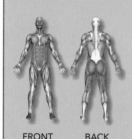

FRONT   BACK

• Abdominals
• Core
• Hamstrings

PLANK LEG EXTENSION

1 In prone position, support your upper body with your hands and keep your arms directly below your shoulders. Your legs should be straight and hip-width apart.

2 Keeping your abs flexed, exhale and raise your right leg, lengthening your body as your weight transfers from your arms to your left foot.

3 Return your right foot to the floor and repeat.

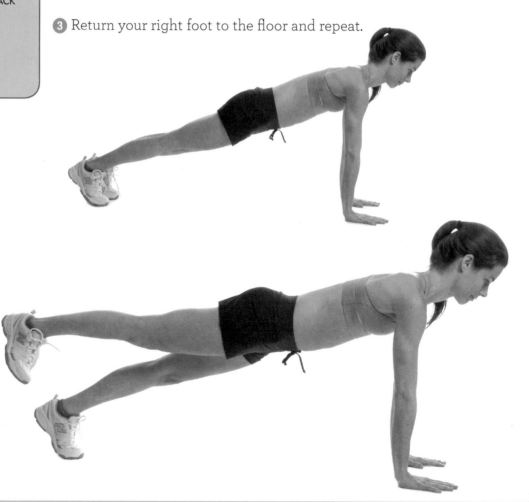

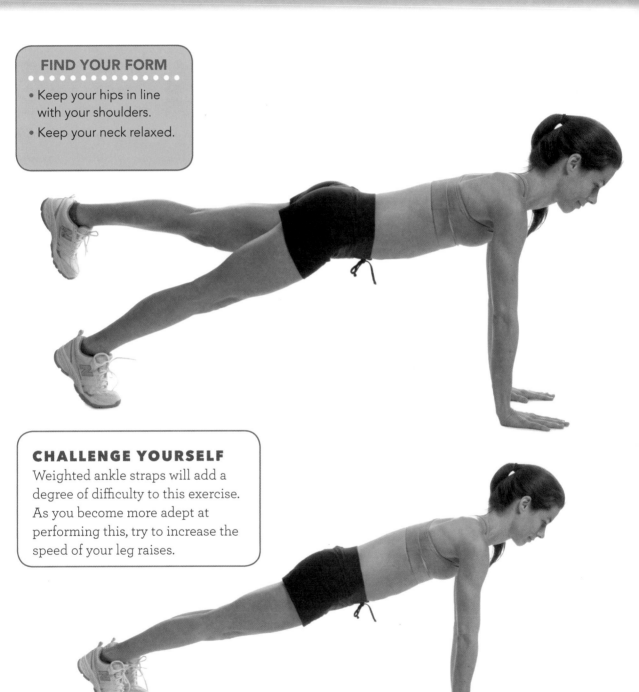

FIND YOUR FORM

• Keep your hips in line with your shoulders.

• Keep your neck relaxed.

CHALLENGE YOURSELF

Weighted ankle straps will add a degree of difficulty to this exercise. As you become more adept at performing this, try to increase the speed of your leg raises.

TIME ELAPSED

• 4 min

BEST FOR

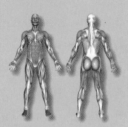

FRONT   BACK

• Abdominals
• Hamstrings
• Shoulders

KETTLEBELL FIGURE 8

1 Assume a wide stance and hold a kettlebell in your right hand, between your legs, close to your right thigh. Bend forwards slightly, keeping your back flat and pushing out your behind.

2 Bring the kettlebell towards your left leg, and receive it in your left hand, which should come from behind the left leg.

3 Repeat the movement with the left hand, giving the kettlebell from in front of the left leg to the right hand behind the right leg. This forms a figure 8 around your static legs.

FIND YOUR FORM

• Keep your back flat throughout the movement.
• Avoid bouncing excessively and relying on momentum.

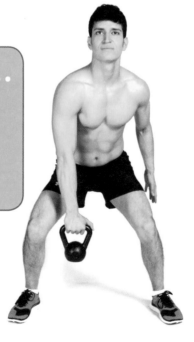

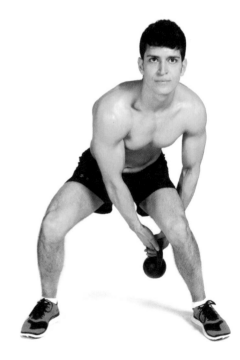

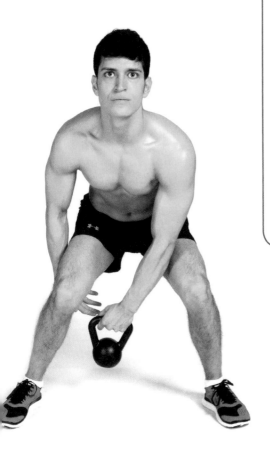

CHALLENGE YOURSELF

Easier: Try the exercise without a kettlebell, just touching hand to hand

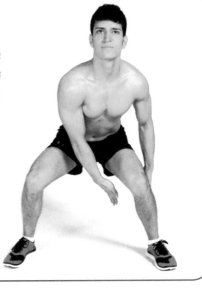

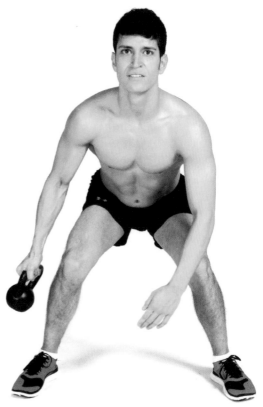

TIME ELAPSED

• 4 min, 30 sec

BEST FOR

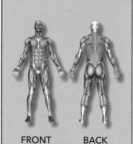

FRONT   BACK

• Back
• Biceps

ALTERNATING KETTLEBELL ROW

1. Stand upright with your feet shoulder-width apart. Hold a pair of kettlebells in front of you with an overhand grip

2. Bend forwards slightly at the waist, maintaining a flat back.

3. Bend your arm at the elbow, and pull your left hand up towards your abdomen, then lower it again.

4. Next, pull your right hand up, then lower it. Complete 8–10 repetitions per hand.

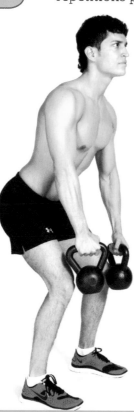

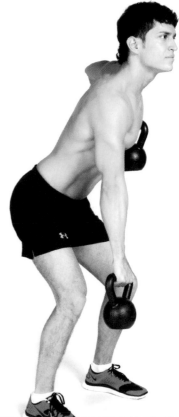

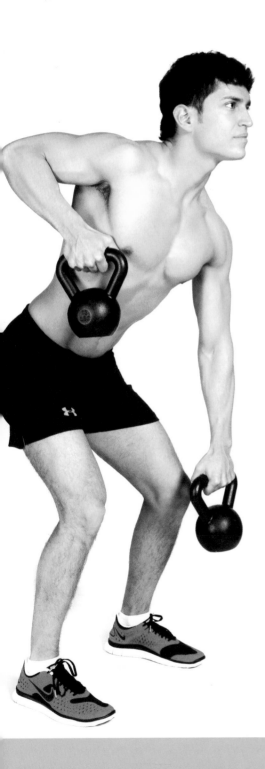

CHALLENGE YOURSELF

Easier: Lift with both arms at the same time.
More difficult: Raise one leg off the floor for a tougher challenge.

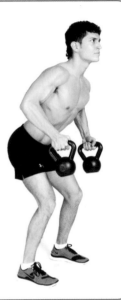

FIND YOUR FORM

- Keep your shoulders and neck relaxed.
- Move your entire body as one unit as you go into the stretch.
- Avoid extending your front knee too far over the planted foot.
- Avoid rotating your hips.
- Avoid shifting your back knee outward.

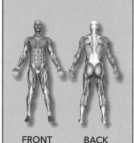
ALTERNATING KETTLEBELL PRESS

1 Stand with your feet shoulder-width apart and a pair of kettlebells cleaned to the sides of your shoulders. Your palms should be facing each other.

2 Raise the right kettlebell directly overhead until your arm locks out, turning the palm forwards in mid-motion. Keep the other kettlebell as still as possible.

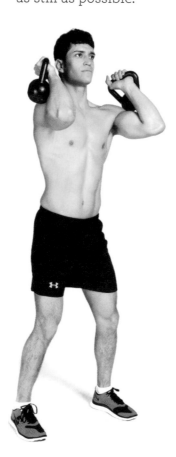

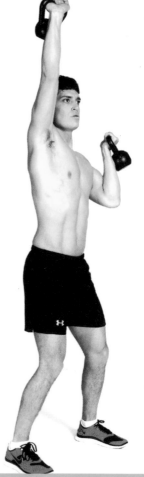

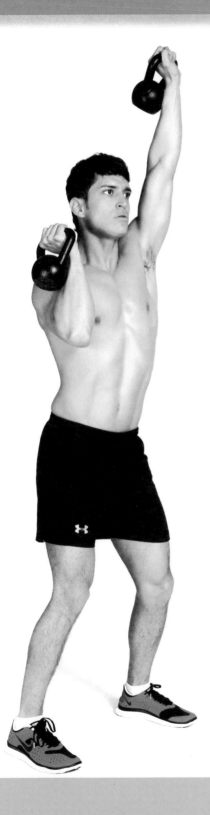

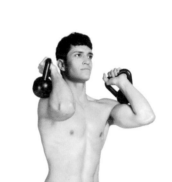

CHALLENGE YOURSELF

Easier: Press with both arms at the same time. More difficult: Raise one leg off the floor for a tougher challenge.

FIND YOUR FORM

- Keep your core engaged and straight on.
- Avoid Leaning back too far when executing the movement.

11

TIME ELAPSED

• 5 min, 30 sec

BEST FOR

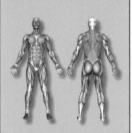

FRONT   BACK

• Back
• Biceps

ONE-ARMED ROW

1 Stand with one leg extended several feet in front of the other, with your front leg bent you're your back heel off the floor. Place one end of your resistance band beneath your front foot and grasp the other end with your opposite hand. Rest your free hand above your knee and lean forward slightly.

2 Bend your arm as you pull the resistance band up toward your chest.

3 Lower and repeat, completing 20 repetitions. Switch sides and repeat.

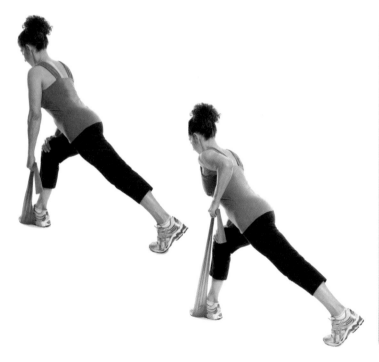

FIND YOUR FORM

• Keep your back flat throughout the exercise.
• Lean forward so that your back leg and your torso form a straight line.
• Move smoothly and in control, engaging your arm muscles.
• Don't allow the end of the resistance band to come loose from beneath your front foot.
• Don't arch your back or neck
• Don't curve your back forwards
• Don't hunch your shoulders
• Don't rush through the movement jerking your arm.

12

TIME ELAPSED

• 6 min

BEST FOR

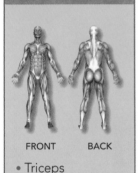

FRONT   BACK

• Triceps

ONE-ARMED TRICEPS KICKBACK

❶ Stand in a lunge position, with your front leg bent and your back heel off the ground. Place one end of the resistance band beneath your front foot and grasp the other end in your opposite hand the other end in your opposite hand.

❷ Lean forward, keeping your back flat so that your torso and back leg form a line. Bend your elbow to position the resistance band next to your hips.

❸ Keep our upper arm in place as you straighten your hand behind you to full lockout.Lower and repeat, performing 15 repetitions. Switch arms and repeat, working up to three sets of 15 per arm.

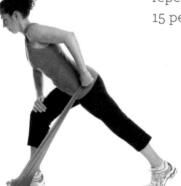

FIND YOUR FORM

• Bend from your hips, not from your waist.
• Try wrapping the resistance band around your front foot.
• Keep your upper arm in place throughout the exercise.
• Rest your free hand above your knee.
• Don't allow the resistance band to come lose from beneath your foot.

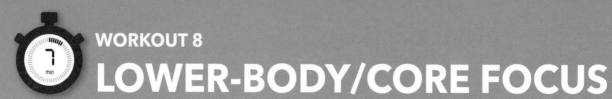

WORKOUT 8

LOWER-BODY/CORE FOCUS

1 Iliotibial Band Stretch

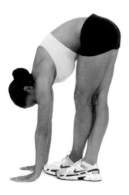

2 Step-Down

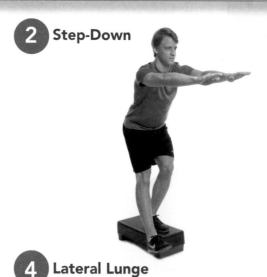

3 Heel-Drop/Toe-Up

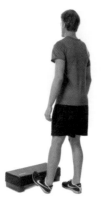

4 Lateral Lunge

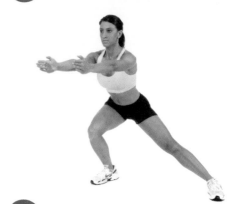

5 Wall Sit

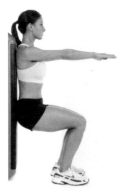

6 Mountain Climber

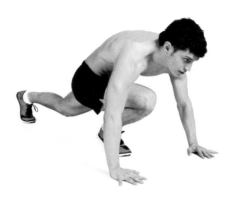

If your goal is to build muscle in your lower body, improve core control and definition, this workout is a good place to start. These exercises are designed to strengthen the muscles in your thighs, glutes, lower back, and abdominals, all of which function in tandem to provide support and stability when performing strenuous workouts. such as lifting weights.

7 Straight-Leg Lunge

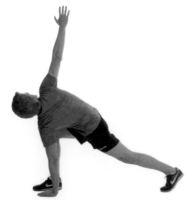

8 Wide-Legged Forward Bend

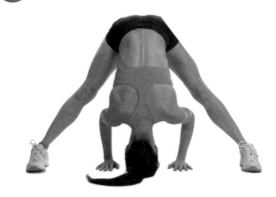

9 Clamshell Series

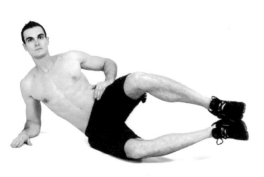

10 Hamstring Flexibility

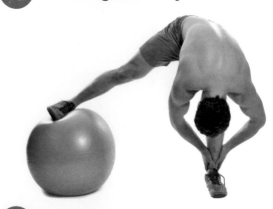

11 Sitting Balance

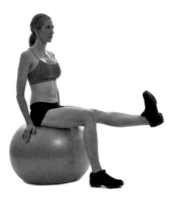

12 Single-Leg Raise

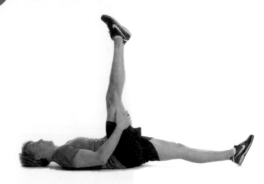

BEST FOR

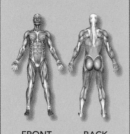

FRONT   BACK

• Hamstrings
• Lower Back

ILIOTIBIAL BAND STRETCH

1 Standing, cross your left leg in front of your right.

2 Bend forward from the hips while keeping both legs straight and reach your hands toward the floor.

3 Hold for several seconds. Repeat the sequence three times on each leg.

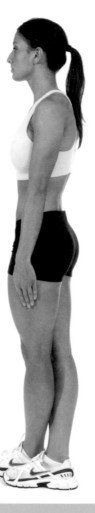

FIND YOUR FORM

• Avoid raising your back heel off the floor
• Avoid arching or round your back.
• Keep both feet flat on the floor.

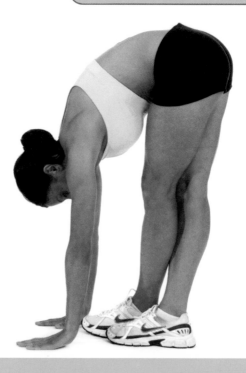

2

TIME ELAPSED

• 1 min

BEST FOR

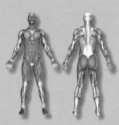

FRONT   BACK

• Thighs
• Core
• Glutes

STEP-DOWN

① Standing up straight on a firm step or block, plant your left foot firmly close to the edge, allowing the right foot to hang off the side. Flex the toes of your right foot.

② Lift your arms out in front of you for balance, keep them parallel to the floor. Lower your torso as you bend at your hips and dropping your right leg towards the floor. Without rotating your knee, press upward through your left leg to return to the starting position. Repeat 15 times for two sets on each leg.

FIND YOUR FORM

• Don't rotate your knee inwards.
• Bend your knees and hips at the same time.
• Keep your hips behind your foot, leaning your torso forwards as you lower into the bend.
• Avoid craning your neck.
• Avoid placing weight on the foot being lowered to the floor.

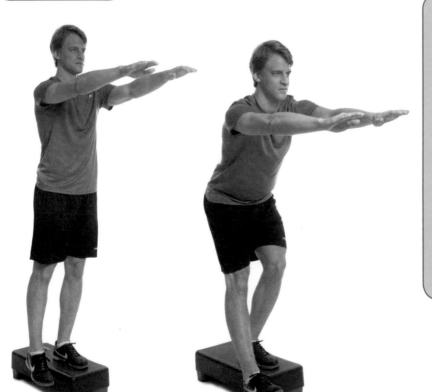

3

TIME ELAPSED

- 1 min, 30 sec

BEST FOR

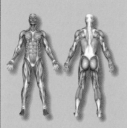

FRONT   BACK

- Hip flexors
- Hip extensors
- Hamstrings
- Quadriceps

HEEL-DROP/TOE-UP

1 Stand on an aerobic step, a block, or a stair with your legs and feet parallel and shoulder width apart. Bend your knees very slightly, keeping your chest up and your shoulders back.

2 Position your left foot slightly in front of your right and place the ball of your right foot on the edge of the step.

3 Drop your right heel down while controlling the amount of weight on the right leg to increase or decrease the intensity of the stretch in the right calf.

4 Release, switch feet and repeat on the other side.

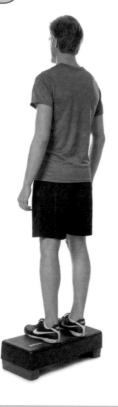

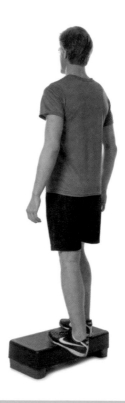

5 Step down from the riser and stand with your legs and feet parallel and shoulder-width apart. Bend your knees very slightly and tuck your pelvis slightly forwards, lift your chest and press your shoulders downwards and back.

6 Position the ball of your left foot on the step.

7 With your knees straight, bring your hips forwards.

8 Release, switch feet and repeat on the other side.

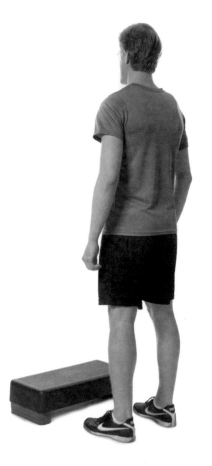

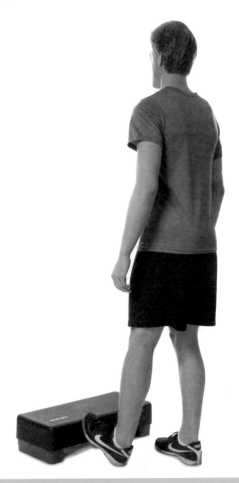

4

TIME ELAPSED

• 2 min

BEST FOR

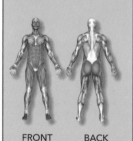

FRONT   BACK

• Glutes
• Thighs
• Core

LATERAL LUNGE

1 Stand with your feet planted widely and your arms outstretched in front of you, parallel to the floor.

2 Step out to the left. Squat down on your right leg, bending at your hips while keeping your back neutral. Begin to extend your left leg, keeping both feet flat on the floor.

3 Bend your right knee until your thigh is parallel to the floor, and your left leg is fully extended.

4 Keeping your arms parallel to the ground, squeeze your buttocks and press off your right leg to return to the starting position, and repeat. Repeat sequence 10 times on each side.

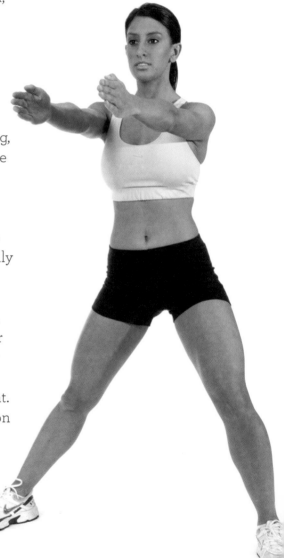

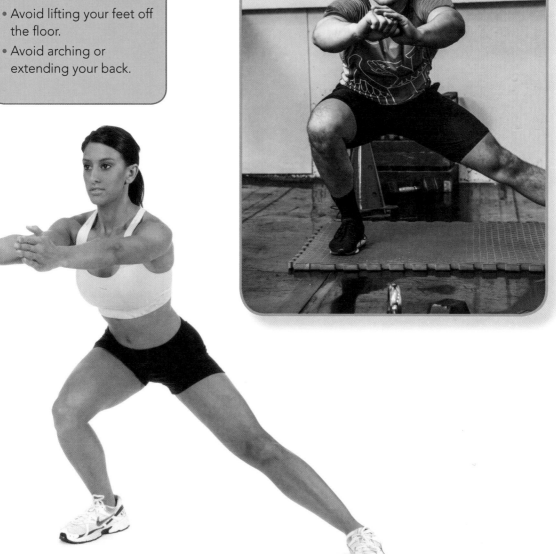

FIND YOUR FORM

- Relax your shoulders and neck.
- Avoid craning your neck as you perform the movement.
- Avoid lifting your feet off the floor.
- Avoid arching or extending your back.

5

BEST FOR

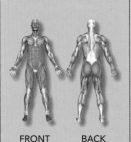

FRONT   BACK

• Glutes
• Thighs
• Core

WALL SIT

1 Stand with your back to a wall. Lean against the wall and walk your feet out from under your body until your lower back rests comfortably against it.

2 Slide your torso down the wall, until your hips and knees form 90-degree angles, your thighs parallel to the floor.

3 Raise your arms straight in front of you so that they are parallel to your thighs and relax the upper torso. Hold for 1 minute, and repeat five times.

FIND YOUR FORM

• Keep your body firm throughout the exercise.
• Relax your shoulders and neck.
• Form a 90-degree angle with your hips and knees.

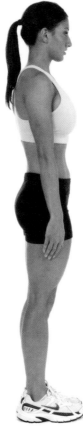

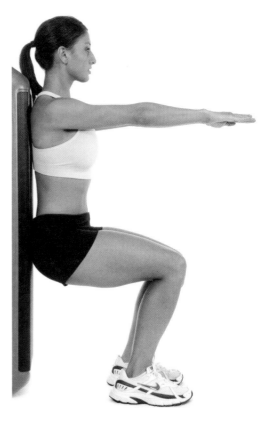

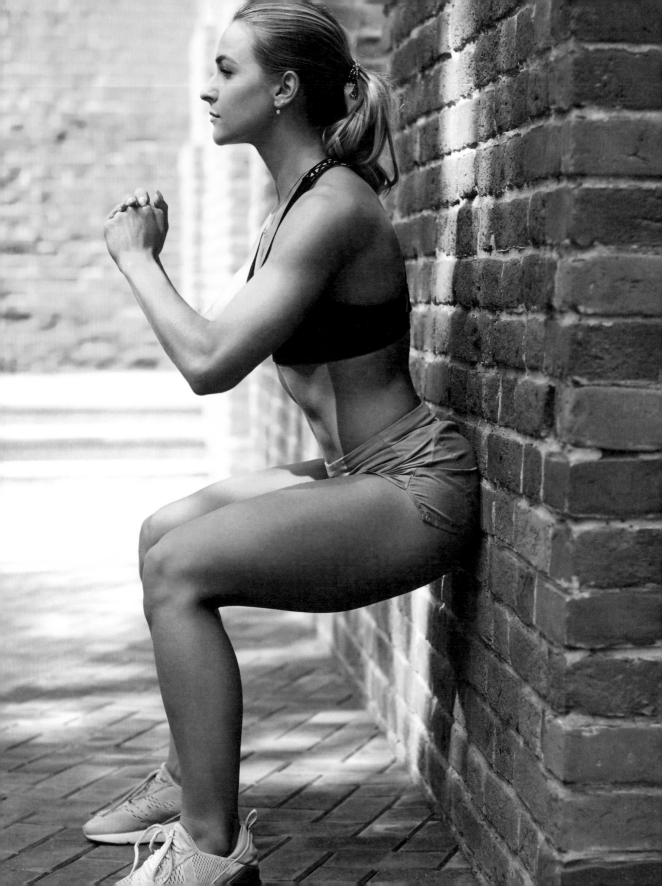

BEST FOR

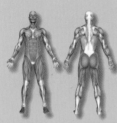

FRONT   BACK

• Glutes
• Thighs
• Hamstrings
• Core

MOUNTAIN CLIMBER

1 Begin in a completed push-up position, with your body in a straight line.

2 Bend one leg and bring your knee as close to your chest as you are able.

3 Return to the starting position and repeat with the other leg.

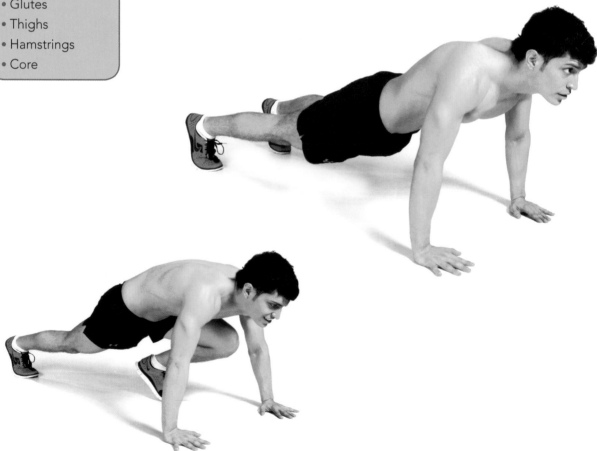

CHALLENGE YOURSELF

More difficult: Wear ankle weights for increased resistance.

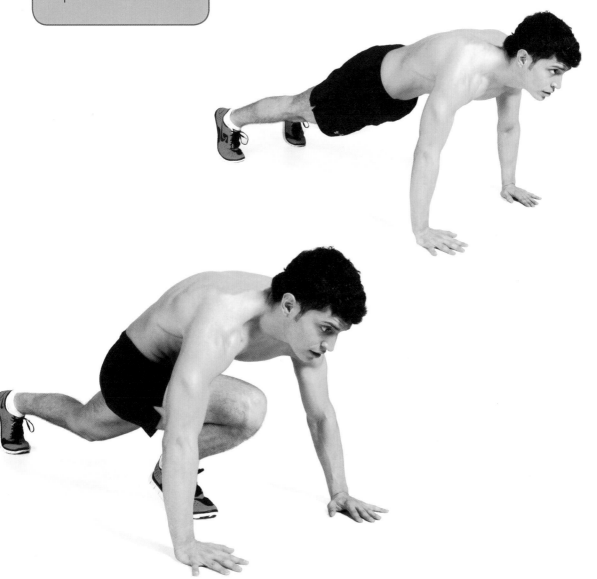

TIME ELAPSED

• 3 min, 30 sec

BEST FOR

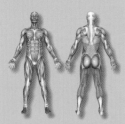

FRONT   BACK

• Hamstrings
• Lower back
• Calves

STRAIGHT-LEG LUNGE

1 Stand with your legs and feet parallel and shoulder width apart. Bend your knees very slightly and tuck your pelvis slightly forwards, lift your chest and press your shoulders downwards and back.

2 Take one step forwards with the right foot.

3 Keeping your legs straight, lean your torso forward over your right leg. Allow the weight of your upper body to intensify the stretch.

4 Return to the starting position and repeat

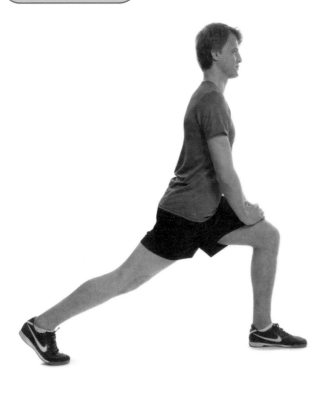

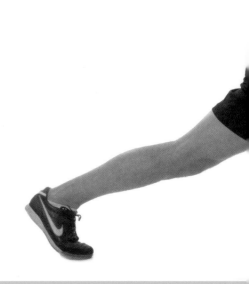

CHALLENGE YOURSELF

Place your hands flat on the floor on either side of the front foot.

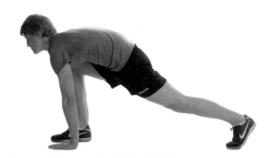

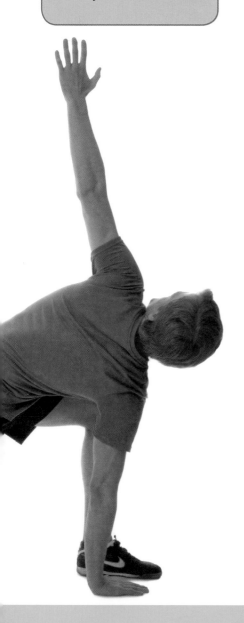

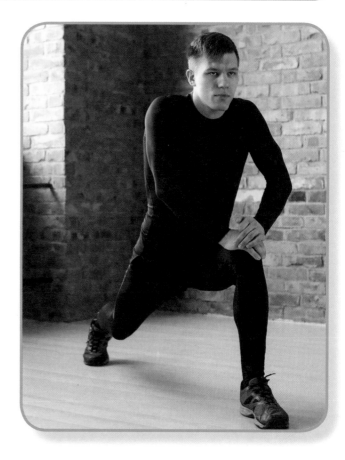

TIME ELAPSED

• 4 min

BEST FOR

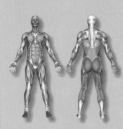

FRONT   BACK

• Hamstrings
• Lower back
• Gluteal area
• Calves

WIDE-LEGGED FORWARD BEND

1 Stand with your legs and feet parallel and wider than shoulder width apart. Bend your knees slightly.

2 Exhale and bend forwards from your hips, keeping your back flat. Draw your sternum forwards as you lower your torso, gazing straight ahead. With your elbows straight, place your fingertips or palms on the floor.

3 With another exhalation, lower to your fullest range of motion, placing your palms on the floor at your feet if possible.

4 Hold for several seconds. To return to your starting position, straighten your elbows and raise your torso while keeping your back flat.

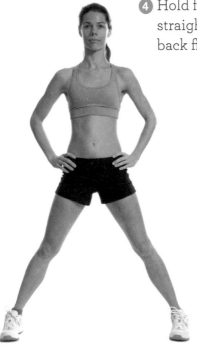

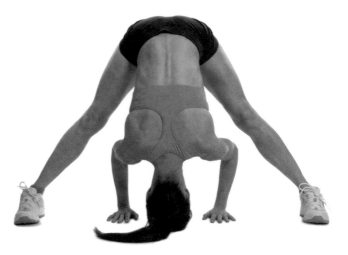

FIND YOUR FORM

- Contract your leg muscles, and keep your feet firmly grounded throughout the stretch.
- Exhale as you hinge forwards from the hips.
- Keep your chest elevated.
- Avoid bending forwards from your waist
- Avoid compressing the back of your neck as you look forwards.
- Avoid tensing your shoulders.

CHALLENGE YOURSELF

Easier: Follow step 1, and then exhale, bending forwards until your torso is nearly parallel to the floor. Place your hands on the floor in line with your shoulders, making sure that your lower back is straight. Hold for several seconds.

Easier: Widen your stance or place a block, book, or other solid object on the floor for support.

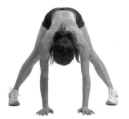 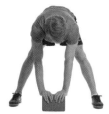

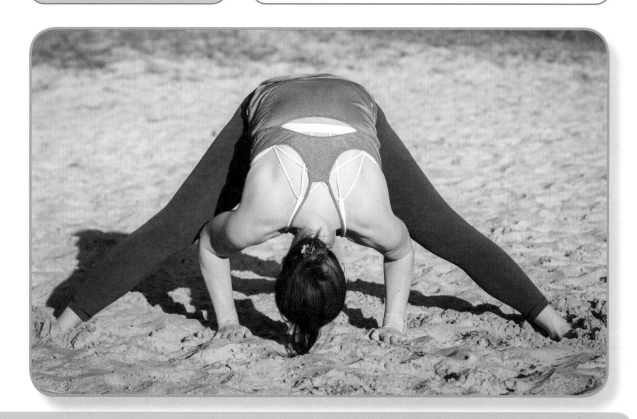

TIME ELAPSED

• 4 min, 30 sec

BEST FOR

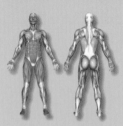

FRONT   BACK

• Abdominals
• Hips
• Thighs

CLAMSHELL SERIES

1 Lie on the ground on your right hip, placing your right forearm on the floor to support yourself. Put your left hand on your left hip. Keep your legs slightly bent, lying one on top of the other.

2 Keeping a straight spine, your right leg on the floor, and your feet together, lift your left knee 10 times.

3 Next, holding your knees and feet together, lift your feet off the floor.

4 While your feet are raised, open and close your knees, again moving only your left leg.

5 Finish step 4 with your knees open, then lift your left leg and straighten it without moving your thigh. Bend your knee again and repeat.

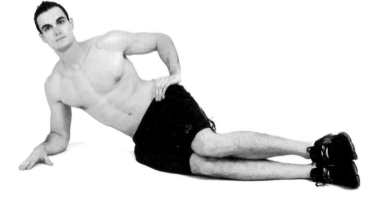

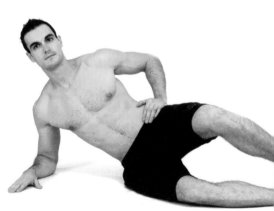

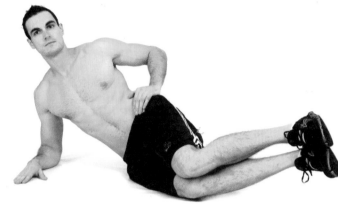

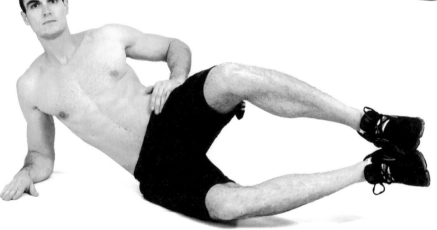

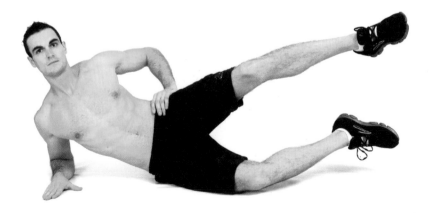

BEST FOR

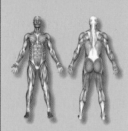

FRONT   BACK

• Hamstrings
• Glutes

HAMSTRING FLEXIBILITY

1 Begin standing on one foot with the other leg outstretched and placed on a Swiss ball to your side.

2 While keeping the supported knee relaxed and your abdominals braced, bend toward your knee and hold for several seconds.

3 Switch sides and repeat.

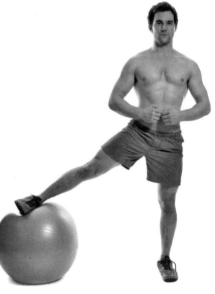

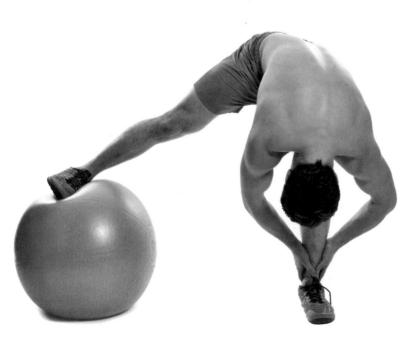

FIND YOUR FORM

• Keep your abdominals braced.
• Keep your knees relaxed
• Move slowly and deliberately.
• Avoid bouncy repetitions.

TIME ELAPSED

• 5 min, 30 sec

BEST FOR

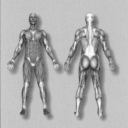

FRONT   BACK

• Abdominals
• Thighs

SITTING BALANCE

1 Sit on a Swiss ball with your feet together and your hands resting on the ball at your sides.

2 Lift one foot off the floor and hold for several seconds.

3 Put your foot down, then lift your other foot.

4 Repeat several times on each leg.

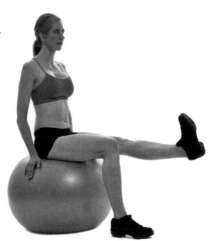

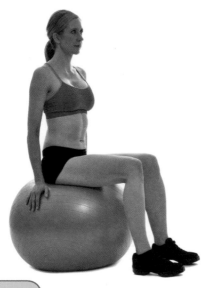

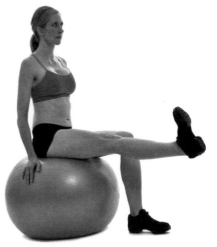

FIND YOUR FORM

• Sit up straight.
• Keep your abdominals activated.
• Avoid leaning forward as you lift your leg

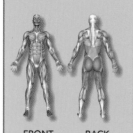
SINGLE-LEG RAISE

1 Lie on your back with both legs extended and your spine in an imprinted position so your lower back touches the floor.

2 With your hands placed on your hamstrings just below the knee, extend and straighten your left leg towards the ceiling.

3 Point both feet and hold for several seconds, then switch legs and repeat on the other side.

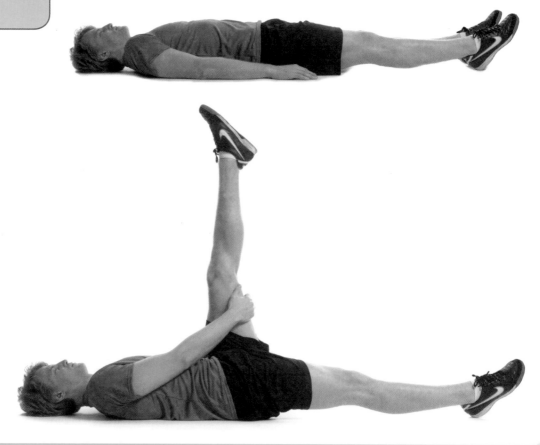

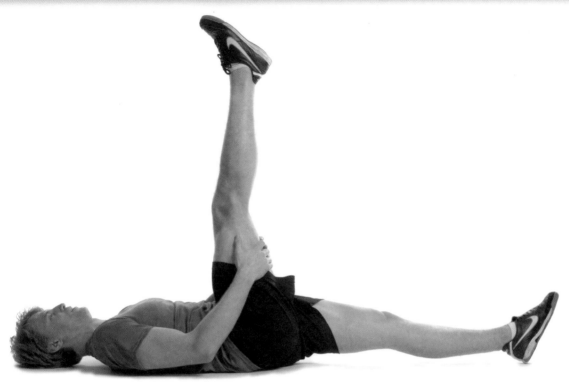

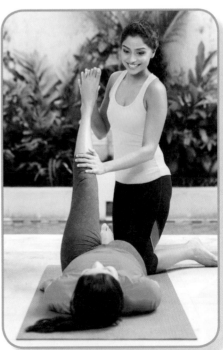

FIND YOUR FORM

• Keep your back and hips flush to the floor.

• Avoid lifting your head or upper back.

• Breathe evenly.

ICON INDEX

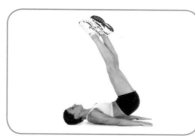

Abdominal Kick
p86-87

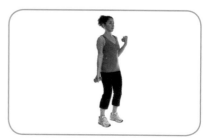

Alternating Hip Lift
p88-89

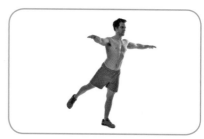

Alternating Dumbbell Curl
p62-63

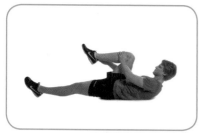

Alternating Kettlebell Press
p158-59

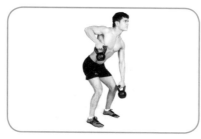

Alternating Kettlebell Row
p156-57

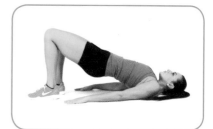

Balance Walk
p126-27

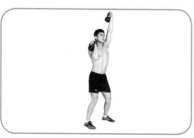

Bench Dip
p38-39

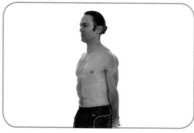

Biceps-Pecs Stretch
p19

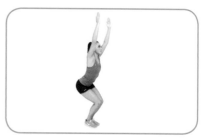

Bridge
p90

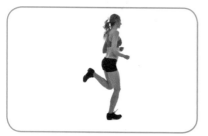

Butt Kicks
p36-37

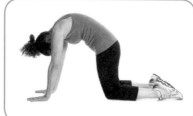

Cat-to Cow
p106-7

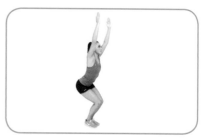

Chair Pose
p116

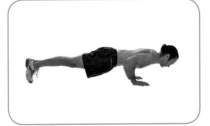

Chaturanga
p101

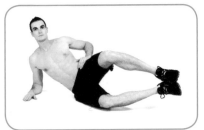

Clamshell Series
p178-79

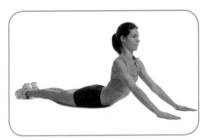

Cobra Stretch
p102-3

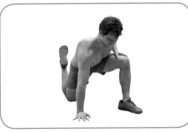

Couch Stretch
p25

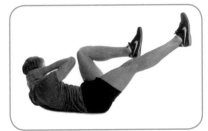

Crossover Crunch
p52-53

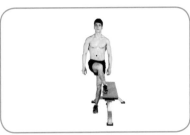

Crossover Step-Up
p54-55

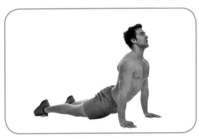

Diver's Push-Up
p50-51

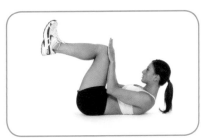

Double-Leg Abdominal Press
p84

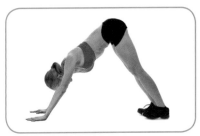

Downward-Facing Dog
p108-9

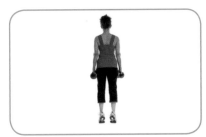

Dumbbell Calf Raise
p73

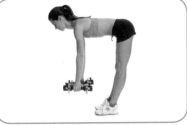

Dumbbell Deadlift
p58-59

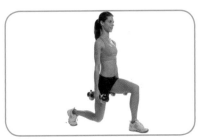

Dumbbell Lunge
p66-67

ICON INDEX

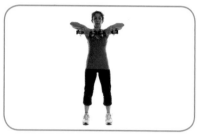

Dumbbell Upright Row
p71

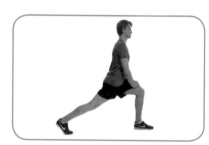

Forward Lunge
p46-47

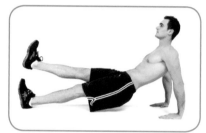

Front Plank
p92-93

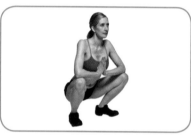

Garland Pose
p114-15

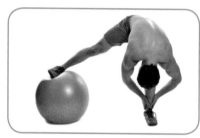

Hamstring Flexibility
p180

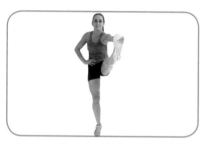

Hand-to-Toe Lift
p132

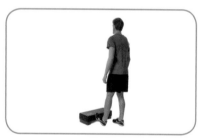

Heel-Drop/Toe-Up
p166-67

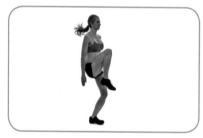

High Knees
p34-35

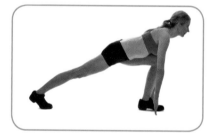

High Lunge
p112-13

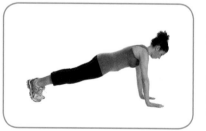

High Plank Pose
p100

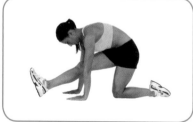

Hip Flexor and Hamstrings Stretch
p22-23

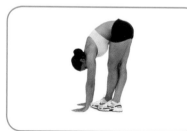

Iliotibial Band Stretch
p164

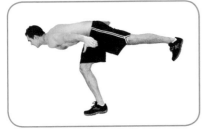
Inverted Hamstring
p128-29

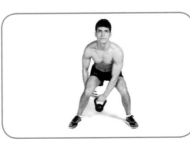
Kettlebell Figure 8
p154-55

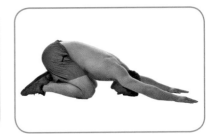
Kneeling Lat Stretch
p31

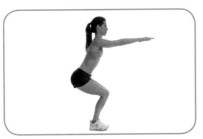
Knee Squat
p133

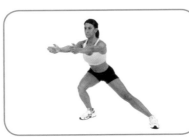
Lateral Lunge
p168-69

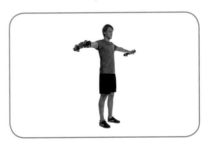
Lateral Shoulder Raise
p68-69

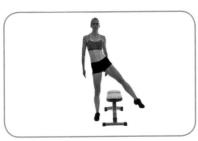
Lateral Stepover
p48-49

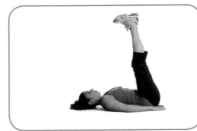
Leg Raise
p85

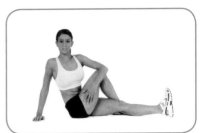
Lower-Back and Hip Stretch
p26

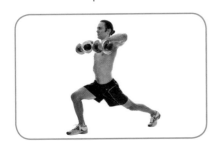
Lunge with Dumbbell Upright Row
p74-75

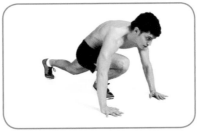
Mountain Climber
p172-73

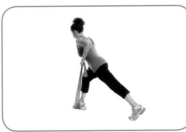
One-Armed Row
p160

ICON INDEX

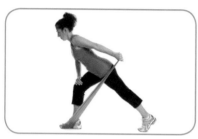

One-Armed Triceps Kickback
p161

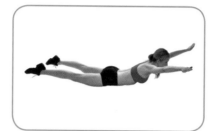

Pilates X
p82-83

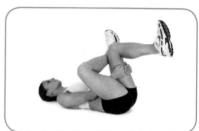

Piriformis Stretch
p30

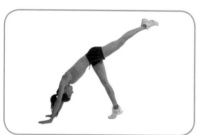

Plank Knee Pull-In
p130-1

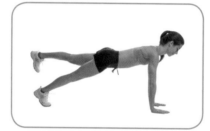

Plank Leg Extension
p152-53

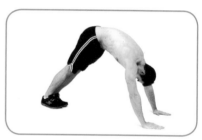

Plank Roll-Down
p110-11

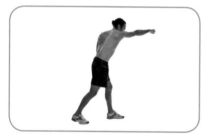

Power Punch
p42

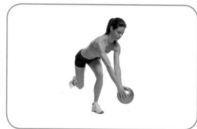

Power Squat
p137

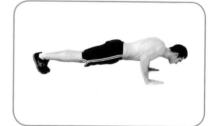

Push-Up
p146-47

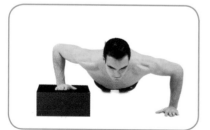

Push-Up Hand Walkover
p150-1

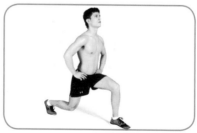

Reverse Lunge
p134-35

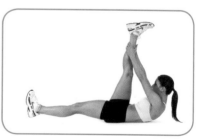

Scissors
p96-97

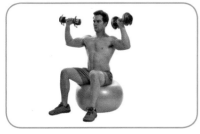

Seated Alternating Dumbbell Press
p76-77

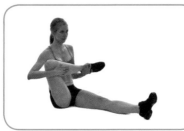

Seated Leg Cradle
p27

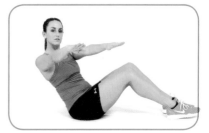

Seated Russian Twist
p142-43

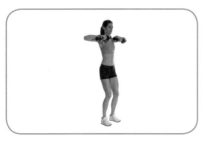

Shoulder Raise and Pull
p70

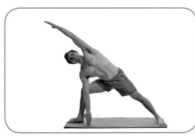

Side-Angle Pose
p118-19

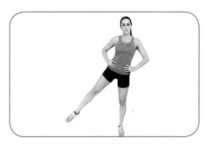

Single-Leg Balance
p124-25

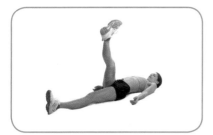

Single-Leg Circles
p94-95

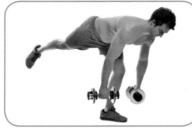

Single-Leg Deadlift
p64-65

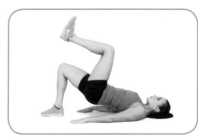

Single-Leg Glute Bridge
p91

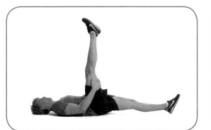

Single-Leg Raise
p182-83

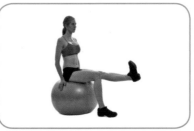

Sitting Balance
p181

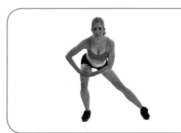

Skater's Lunge
p40-41

ICON INDEX

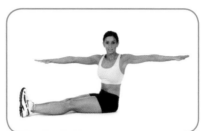

Spine Stretch
p28-29

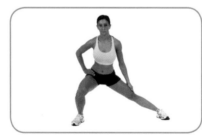

Spine Twist
p80

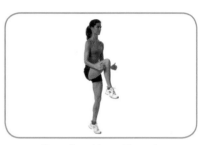

Standing Knee Crunch
p136

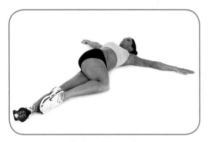

Standing Stability
p123

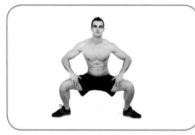

Static Sumo Squat
p122

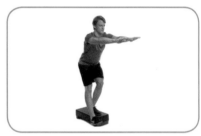

Step-Down
p165

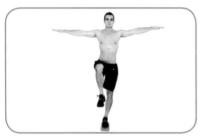

Step-Up
p44-45

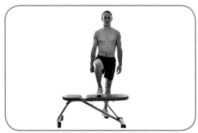

Straddle Abductor Stretch
p21

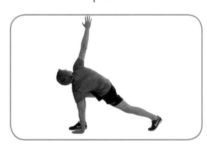

Straight-Leg Lunge
p174-75

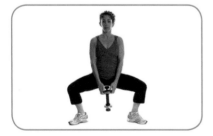

Sumo Squat
p72

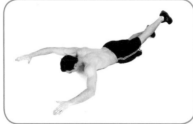

Swimming
p144

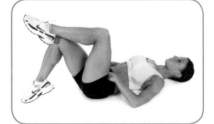

Tiny Steps
p81

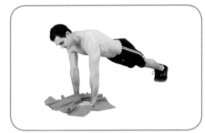

Towel Fly
p145

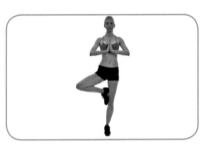

Tree Pose
p117

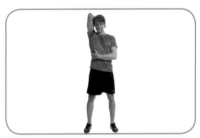

Triceps Extension
p60-61

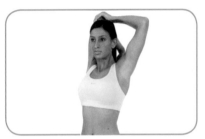

Triceps Stretch
p20

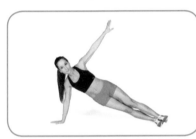

T-Stabilization
p148-49

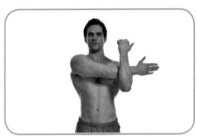

Upper-Back / Shoulder Stretch
p18

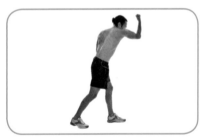

Uppercut
p43

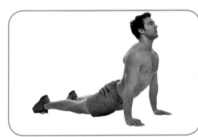

Upward-Facing Dog
p104-5

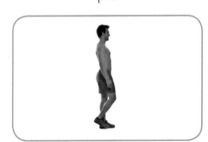

Walking Heel-to-Toe
p138-39

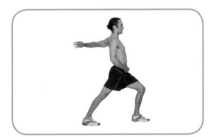

Wall-Assisted Chest Stretch
p24

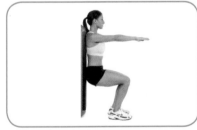

Wall Sit
p170-1

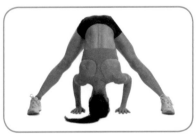

Wide-Legged Forward Bend
p176-77

CREDITS

All exercise models in this book are from moseleyroad.inc.
For any individual model information, please contact: amoore@moseleyroad.com

All other images are from shuttterstock.
p9 Jacob Lund. p11 VGstockstudio. p13 KlaraBstock. p29 fizkes. p35 bbernard. p41 puhhha. p47 Sjale.
p59 Undrey. p63 Jacob Lund. p67 wavebreakmedia. p83 Maridav. p103 Khrystyna Bohush. p105,7&9 fizkes. p115 Mindful Media Creations.
p131 Anna Berdnick. p135 sakkmesterke. p147 Master 1305. p149 fizkes. p169 Ivan Kulezic. p171 The Faces.
p175 Y Studio. p177 Fotographie. p183 Kzenon.